The Mental Status Examination in Neurology

Third Edition

The Mental Status Examination in Neurology

Third Edition

Richard L. Strub, MD
Chairman
Department of Neurology
Ochsner Clinic
Clinical Professor of Neurology
Tulane University
New Orleans, Louisiana

F. William Black, PhD
Professor of Psychiatry and Neurology
Director, Neuropsychology Laboratory
Tulane University Medical Center
New Orleans, Louisiana

Foreword by Norman Geschwind

 F. A. DAVIS COMPANY • Philadelphia

F. A. Davis Company
1915 Arch Street
Philadelphia, PA 19103

Printed in the United States of America

Last digit indicates print number: 10 9 8 7 6 5 4

Acquisitions Editor: Robert H. Craven, Sr.
Medical Developmental Editor: Bernice M. Wissler
Production Editor: Crystal S. McNichol
Cover Design by: Steven R. Morrone

As new scientific information becomes available through basic and clinical research, recommended treatments and drug therapies undergo changes. The author(s) and publisher have done everything possible to make this book accurate, up to date, and in accord with accepted standards at the time of publication. The authors, editors, and publisher are not responsible for errors or omissions or for consequences from application of the book, and make no warranty, expressed or implied, in regard to the contents of the book. Any practice described in this book should be applied by the reader in accordance with professional standards of care used in regard to the unique circumstances that may apply in each situation. The reader is advised always to check product information (package inserts) for changes and new information regarding dose and contraindications before administering any drug. Caution is especially urged when using new or infrequently ordered drugs.

Library of Congress Cataloging-in-Publication Data
Strub, Richard L., 1939-
 The mental status examination in neurology / Richard L. Strub, F. William Black ; foreword by Norman Geschwind. — 3rd ed.
  p. cm.
 Includes bibliographical references and index.
 ISBN 0-8036-8212-3 (softback : alk. paper)
  1. Mental status examination. 2. Neurobehavioral disorders—Diagnosis. I. Black, F. William. II. Title.
  [DNLM: 1. Nervous System Diseases—diagnosis. 2. Neurologic Examination.
WL 141 S925m 1993]
RC386.6,M44S87 1993
616.85′884—dc20
DNLM/DLC
for Library of Congress   93-18229
                                                                                  CIP

In memory of Dr. Norman Geschwind, 1926–1984

Foreword

The testing of mental status has a curious, not to say anomalous, position in the examination of patients. Every medical student has had the experience of being given a long and detailed outline, or an even longer booklet, containing a seemingly endless list of items. Even if he should go to the trouble of memorizing these miniature compendia, he is likely to discover that his teachers, both neurologic and psychiatric, are disinclined to be concerned with the detailed examination, and often rely, at best, on fragments. The examinations themselves seem to differ from those in other fields of medicine. The student rapidly comes to appreciate the direct relevance of rectal tenderness to the diagnosis of appendicitis or of pulsus paradoxus to pericardial effusion. The mental examination seems to him to be much more indirectly and diffusely related to diagnostic categories.

Equally striking, or even more so, is the usual lack of direct correlation between the test items and disorders of structure or physiology. Orthopnea, swollen neck veins, rales at the lung bases, cardiac enlargement, characteristic murmurs, and auricular fibrillation not only mean congestive failure, but all the findings on examination come to blend almost imperceptibly and effortlessly with knowledge of normal cardiac structures and physiology and awareness of lawful derangements in disease. This easy understanding of the relationship of abnormal findings on examination to anatomy and physiology seems to be lacking in the mental examination.

There is, however, no reason that this situation should persist. The growth of knowledge concerning disorders of the higher functions has been rapid over the past quarter century. Not only has our ability to specify anatomic systems involved in different behaviors increased, but even more important, we have come to a deeper understanding of the mechanisms underlying disordered function.

This book, therefore, represents a valuable synthesis. For the attentive reader, it will yield important advantages. Not only does it shift the emphasis to those methods of examination that have proven their worth in the clinic but it provides wherever possible a link to known anatomic and physiologic mechanisms.

Several final comments are appropriate. There is a widespread, usually tacit but often openly expressed, view that mental examination is a long and arduous task. Most physicians have learned that although a "complete" survey of the heart, lungs, abdomen, and other structures can take hours, intimate knowledge of the examination and repeated practice enable them to obtain essential information in a very brief time. Those who have learned the mental examination and have practiced it often can equally well obtain vital information rapidly and efficiently when necessary. There is another common view that mental examination can be handed over to others. We should remember, however, that the real measure of a physician's usefulness lies in his capacity to make critical decisions when he is alone with the patient in the small hours of the night. Furthermore, unless he can screen patients effectively, he will fail to refer intelligently to others. Finally, if the ultimate decisions lie in his hands, he will fail to use adequately the opinions of his consultants unless he has a basic understanding of all aspects of his patient's problems. The newer knowledge of mental examination set forth within this book is essential not merely to the neurologist or psychiatrist, but to all physicians.

Norman Geschwind, MD
James Jackson Putnam Professor of Neurology
Harvard Medical School
1977

Preface

The basic purpose and scope of this book have not changed since the first edition was published in 1977. In the intervening years, we have gained considerable additional clinical experience with the mental status examination and have standardized most sections of the examination. Some of the standardized items have been compared with the objective data generated from formal neuropsychologic tests. These comparisons have been very rewarding, as the mental status examination has proven to be an accurate and valid method for identifying and diagnosing organic brain disease, as well as for describing relative levels of functioning. Age-related norms are presented for most aspects of the examination. These data are important because we have found that our patients aged 70 and older do perform less adequately than the younger patients on some of the critical items, especially new learning. This is important to take into account when assessing the elderly for early dementia. False positive results can occur and must be minimized.

In the first edition, we assured the reader that after reading and using the book, he or she would be able to perform a brief screening examination. It has been suggested that we provide more concrete guidelines for tailoring the examination for brief administration. Therefore, in the summary section of this edition, we have included some ways to use the examination as a screening procedure, particularly in the extremely important areas of diagnosing dementia and differentiating between organic and functional disorders. A shortened form of the examination is presented with standardization for normals of various ages and patients with Alzheimer's disease.

We have updated the references in all chapters; this is particularly true in those sections in which new studies have refined the neuroanatomic and neuropsychologic aspects of cognitive functions. The section on neuropsychologic testing has been fully revised to include a survey of the most commonly used tests, to drop some tests that have fallen from general use, and to make this section more clinically relevant to both physicians and psychologists.

In general, we feel that the earlier editions were good and have demonstrated their value in widespread clinical use. The third edition is better, however, because we have now refined and standardized the examination. We hope this text will prove as useful to others who are interested in neurobehavior as it has been to our students, residents, and professional colleagues.

R. L. Strub, MD
F. W. Black, PhD

Contents

Chapter 1

The Mental Status Examination: A Rationale and Overview

Human behavior is extremely complex and multifaceted. Because of its complexity, it is not surprising that brain disease or dysfunction can significantly affect a patient's behavior. Understanding this behavioral disruption in brain disease is a substantial and often frustrating problem to the clinician who is faced with the tasks of diagnosis and management. Patients with organically related changes in cognitive or emotional behavior unfortunately have often fallen just outside the limits of both psychiatry and neurology. Behavior problems within this relatively uncharted borderland have long been considered organic brain syndromes, a general term that covers any possible behavior change resulting from brain damage or dysfunction. In the latest edition of the American Psychiatric Association's *Diagnostic and Statistical Manual of Mental Disorders* (DSM-III-R),[1] such conditions are categorized as organic mental disorders. The DSM-III-R makes a distinction between an organic brain syndrome, which refers to a general clinical constellation of behavioral signs and symptoms (e.g., delirium or dementia), and an organic mental disorder, which denotes a specific disease entity such as Alzheimer's dementia or an amnesic syndrome secondary to head trauma. This diagnostic scheme is being reviewed and may change in the near future. The new, comprehensive term for these conditions now under consideration by the American Psychiatric Association is *cognitive disorders.*[4] Neurologists now use the term *neurobehavioral disorders.*

In recent years, there has been a renewed interest in these organic syndromes. It is now possible, owing to a greater understanding of these conditions, to relate specific patterns of behavioral deficits to specific diseases and to damage in particular regions of the brain.

The study of neurobehavioral disorders has now reached the same stage of medical popularity as arteriosclerotic heart disease, cancer, and the autoimmune disorders. The magnitude and social impact of these conditions is finally being realized. These disorders are very common in the hospital and office practices of primary care physicians as well as those of neurologists and psychiatrists. Dementia, aphasia, and confusional states (delirium) are not rare conditions that medical students dutifully learn about in medical school and then fruitlessly search for in clinical

1

practice. Quite the opposite is true: these are problems that the average clinician sees every day. Primary organic brain disease accounted for at least 30% of all first admissions to psychiatric hospitals in the 1950s,[2] and this incidence is increasing.[3] Dementia is now the fourth leading cause of death in the adult population in this country, a trend that can only worsen as the lifespan increases. Students should now recognize signs of early dementia as readily as they do those of acquired immune deficiency syndrome (AIDS) or congestive heart failure.

For examiners to understand adequately organically based behavior change and to apply this understanding to individual clinical cases, they must use a systematic behavioral examination. This evaluation, the mental status examination, is an orderly assessment of the important cognitive and emotional functions that are commonly and characteristically disturbed in patients with organic brain disease.

Because the mental status examination is not always included in a routine neurologic evaluation, it is important that the clinician be able to determine when inclusion of the mental status examination is appropriate. Just as the patient with otitis externa does not routinely require an electrocardiogram, the patient with a peripheral neuropathy does not usually need a full mental status examination. Conversely, any patient who complains of memory difficulty should have a comprehensive mental status examination, just as the patient with a fever, headache, and stiff neck requires an immediate computed tomography (CT) scan and lumbar puncture.

There are many patients for whom full mental status testing is definitely indicated. Patients with known brain lesions such as tumors, trauma, or vascular accident should have an initial screening mental status evaluation to document any cognitive or emotional changes. Even with the current state of neurobehavioral knowledge, subtle (and even gross) behavioral deficits secondary to brain lesions are sometimes overlooked or considered inconsequential by the treating physician. Many patients with mild aphasias or memory deficits after craniotomy, increased irritability and decreased ability to concentrate after head trauma, or marked emotional lability after infectious neurologic disease are released from the hospital without adequate recognition of these cognitive and emotional deficits. Such patients frequently become emotionally frustrated, have difficulty with social readjustment, and are unable to carry out the routine demands of home and vocation. Early recognition of these neurobehavioral sequelae of known neurologic disorders helps the physician explain the totality of the patient's disability to the family and employers. This prevents needless frustration on the patient's part, as well as misunderstanding of the patient's behavior by family members. Such documentation helps immeasurably in planning social and vocational rehabilitation when indicated.

Another large group of patients in whom mental status testing is indicated are those in whom a brain lesion is suspected because of recent onset of seizures, headaches, behavior change, or head trauma. Brain tumors, subdural hematomas, small infarcts, or cerebral atrophy may go undetected on the routine neurologic examination, whereas the cognitive effects of these lesions are often readily apparent on a complete mental status examination. Thus, the inclusion of the mental status examination as an integral component of the initial neurologic evaluation may significantly increase the probability of detecting neurologic disease when present and effectively rule it out when absent. We have seen a 46-year-old man who was admitted to the infectious disease isolation unit because of fever, jumbled speech, and confusion. His admitting diagnosis was "probable encephalitis." Mental status testing the morning after admission revealed an aphasia rather than a confusional state. Because the finding of aphasia is almost pathognomonic of significant left hemisphere disease, a left carotid arteriogram was performed and a large subdural hematoma found. With appropriate treatment (surgery), the patient had an uneventful and complete recovery. Had the correct diagnosis not been made quickly, the patient could well have died without appropriate treatment and with the incorrect diagnosis of "devastating herpes simplex encephalitis." Because of the widespread use of noninvasive neuroimaging techniques, particularly CT and magnetic resonance imaging (MRI), it is much less likely now that a mass lesion would remain undetected in such a setting, but in patients in whom the diagnosis of neurologic disease is equivocal, the mental status examination can be as specific in documenting a brain lesion and indicating its location as the elicitation of Babinski's sign.

A full mental status examination should be performed on all psychiatric patients, particularly those whose psychiatric symptoms have appeared rather acutely and are superimposed on a life history of normal emotional functioning. Patients with organic brain disease frequently initially present with emotional and behavioral changes and come first to the attention of the family physician or consulting psychiatrist.[3] This presentation is especially characteristic of frontal and temporal tumors, hydrocephalus, or cortical atrophy.

The most common emotional change seen in such patients is depression; therefore, brain disease should be strongly suspected in any patient with a middle- or late-life depression that is not clearly related to a recent emotional or social crisis (i.e., adjustment disorder with depressed mood). In our clinical practice, we have seen a large number of patients who were being treated with psychotropic drugs, psychotherapy, electroshock, or long-term psychiatric hospitalization for an apparent depressive illness who have, in fact, demonstrated clear signs of primary organic disease on mental status testing and subsequent neurodiagnostic procedures (e.g., CT and MRI and neuropsychologic evaluation). It is far more economic, efficacious, and appropriate to spend 15 minutes of the initial interview doing a complete mental status examination than to embark on a lengthy, expensive, and sometimes inappropriate treatment regimen.

The differentiation between psychiatric and organic diseases is critically important, but unfortunately sometimes difficult and not always possible. The functionally depressed patient with psychomotor retardation may perform poorly on some aspects of the mental status examination and in this way superficially present the picture of a true dementia rather than a pseudodementia. Other patients have elements of both organic and functional disease; for example, patients with early Alzheimer's dementia often present with significant associated depression or anxiety. At times, considerable effort is required to separate the respective components, even on careful clinical examination. The mental status examination is not infallible, even in the hands of an experienced examiner. The fact remains, however, that the majority of such patients with combined problems can be correctly classified if appropriate mental testing is done.

A final group of patients in whom mental status screening is extremely important is those who initially present, or are brought in by their families, with vague behavioral complaints that are difficult clinically to substantiate and quantify on standard neurologic examination.

Complaints such as memory problems, difficulty in concentration, declining interest in family or work, or a variety of physical complaints without obvious organic etiology should alert the clinician to the possibility of organic brain disease. The determination of the etiology of such problems involves a difficult but important differentiation among functional, neurologic, and other medical causes. Again, this can often be best accomplished with the aid of data provided by the mental status examination.

Mental status testing must be arranged in a systematic fashion. In this sense, the examination is analogous to any comprehensive medical examination. The mental status examination does differ somewhat in that it must be performed in a hierarchical manner, beginning with the most basic function—level of consciousness—and proceeding through the basic cognitive functions (e.g., language, constructions) to the more complex areas of verbal reasoning and calculating ability.

When the patient shows impaired performance on early sections of the examination (e.g., in language), it will be difficult, if not impossible, for the examiner to assess accurately verbal memory (an extremely important function) or any other function that requires language. Similarly, the patient who is inattentive will miss important details during much of the higher-level testing, especially on memory and calculation items. If the mental status examination is performed in a haphazard manner, without regard for the hierarchic nature of cognitive performance, erroneous conclusions will be drawn. The examination must be performed in an orderly way, assessing basic processes first and the higher-level functions such as abstract reasoning subsequently.

The mental status examination as presented in this book may seem exceptionally detailed, and it may appear that the examination would take hours to complete in its entirety. This conception is similar to the beginning clinician's first attempts to understand the evaluation of the cranial nerves or the brachial plexus. When first learning to administer the examination, it is wise to evaluate several patients fully to gain experience in performing and interpreting all test items. With time, the examination can be completed relatively rapidly (within 15 to 30 minutes) and will yield considerable valuable data. In Chapter 10, we have summarized the examination and indicated how it can be tailored to meet the demands of time and the particular patient.

In many cases, a brief examination will provide sufficient definitive data to allow the correct diagnosis and appropriate medical treatment. As an example of the ease of administering a meaningful examination in a brief period of time, a psychiatrist, called in the middle of the night to see a patient who was "talking out of his head," started to examine the patient's language and found that the patient was actually aphasic and not psychotic. At this point, the psychiatrist consulted with a neurologist, who admitted the patient to the neurology service rather than to the psychiatric unit. In this case, the psychiatrist had properly evaluated the patient and averted an inappropriate type of hospitalization and treatment. We were called to see a similar case, in which a young man had been admitted to the psychiatric service because he was answering all questions inappropriately and did not make sense in conversation. This behavior had initially disturbed his parents, who had brought him to the emergency room. On evaluation, the patient had little, if any, comprehension of language and was producing fluent paraphasic speech (aphasia). An MRI scan revealed a large hematoma in the dominant temporal lobe. His apparent "craziness" was due to a readily diagnosed organic disorder, and his psychiatric hospitalization had resulted from the admitting physician's lack of recognition of the patient's actual condition. In this case, demonstration of a typical pattern of aphasia not only indicated the presence of organic disease, but also strongly suggested the location of the lesion.

These examples illustrate that even a brief examination in the hands of a skilled examiner can be of critical clinical importance. In other patients a more comprehensive assessment is required. The patient who is referred after a head injury requires a detailed elucidation of cognitive strengths and deficits to allow for appropriate social and vocational rehabilitation. This need for a comprehensive mental status examination is amply demonstrated in the following case. The physical medicine service requested a consultation on a 32-year-old woman who had suffered a severe basilar skull fracture several months previously and was not progressing satisfactorily in the inpatient rehabilitation program. The staff also noted her "difficult" and "uncooperative" behavior. Mental status testing revealed an apathetic patient without insight or concern, who had moderately impaired attention and vigilance. Multiple significant cognitive deficits were demonstrated, including a mild generalized dementia, moderately impaired recent and remote memory, severely impaired new-learning ability, and a moderate to severe impairment of all higher-level cognitive functions (abstraction, calculations, and so forth). The documentation of an organic behavior change and significant cognitive deficits explained both the patient's difficult ward behavior and her inability to participate fully in a demanding rehabilitation program. Her program was restructured and her treatment goals were altered because of the limitations caused by the cognitive and behavioral deficits.

In complicated situations, when extensive and quantitative data regarding cognitive and emotional functioning are required for proper patient management, consultation should be obtained from relevant ancillary professionals. These frequently include neuropsychologists and speech pathologists. The bedside or office mental status examination as outlined in this book is very effective for diagnosing organic disease and for evaluating major areas of deficit. By its nature, the examination is qualitative and does not offer the advantages of standardized quantitative data, which are necessary in evaluating subtle deficits, planning for comprehensive rehabilitation efforts, and assessing improvements in levels of functioning. The neuropsychologist can provide these data and additional valuable consultation whenever a definitive evaluation is required. Discharge planning and vocational or educational re-entry are also greatly aided by the findings of a comprehensive neuropsychologic assessment.

In patients with significant communication problems, referral to the speech pathologist for comprehensive evaluation of language, possible treatment, and counseling to facilitate communication between the patient and other family members is important. Chapter 11 deals in detail with the specifics of the consultation process. Every clinician should be aware of the availability and scope of such ancillary services and should use them when appropriate to benefit the patient.

REFERENCES

1. American Psychiatric Association: Diagnostic and Statistical Manual of Mental Disorders, ed 3 revised (DSM-III-R). American Psychiatric Association, Washington, DC, 1987.
2. Malzberg, B: Important statistical data about mental illness. In Arieti, S (ed): American Handbook of Psychiatry, Vol 1. Basic Books, New York, 1959, pp 161–174.
3. Strub, RL: Mental disorders in brain disease. In Vinken PJ, Bruyn, GW, and Klawans, HL (eds): Handbook of Clinical Neurology, Vol 2, Neurobehavioral Disorders. Elsevier, New York, 1985, pp 413–441.
4. Tucker, GJ, Caine, ED, Folstein, MF, et al: Introduction to background papers for suggested changes to DSM-IV: Cognitive disorders. Journal of Neuropsychiatry and Clinical Neurosciences 4:360–368, 1992.

Chapter 2

History and Behavioral Observations

Most sections of the mental status examination involve the evaluation of specific cognitive functions such as memory and language. Before beginning formal testing, however, the examiner must take a careful history and make specific and systematic observations of the patient's physical appearance, mood, and behavior. These observations provide information that is important for the interpretation of the data from subsequent parts of the examination.

HISTORY

The history should be directed toward four primary areas of clinical concern. First, the presence or absence of the classic behavioral changes indicative of organic dysfunction (e.g., memory impairment or language disorder) must be established. Second, the possibility of functional psychiatric disorders must be considered. Although this book is primarily concerned with the changes in emotions and behavior that are seen as a result of organic brain disease, the consideration of classic psychiatric syndromes is important for several specific reasons:

1. At times, a specific lesion of the brain (e.g., a tumor of the left frontal lobe) may produce a clinical picture that is indistinguishable from that of a major functional illness.[20,21] Diagnoses of depression or mania, schizophrenia, and personality disorders have all been described as organic brain disease. These are classified in the DSM-III-R[1] as organic affective syndrome, organic delusional syndrome, and organic personality syndrome, respectively.
2. Patients with primary organic disease also commonly develop associated or secondary emotional symptoms such as depression, paranoia, or anxiety.
3. Another important area of overlap between the symptomatology of organic disease and that of emotional disorders is in pseudodementia, a condition in which the patient has symptoms and mental status findings that initially suggest a diagnosis of dementia but eventually prove to be secondary to depression, anxiety, or other psychiatric disorders.

4. Some patients with a major psychiatric disease (e.g., schizophrenia) will demonstrate cognitive deficits on the mental status examination. This may be due to a concomitant acquired brain lesion or may, in fact, be a part of the total clinical picture of these diseases. The incidence of cognitive dysfunction in nonfamilial schizophrenic patients is substantially higher than expected. When significant cognitive deficits are found in psychiatric patients, the appropriate neurodiagnostic procedures should be conducted.

The third focus of the history is to establish the patient's premorbid behavior and level of functioning. Information such as education and vocational history are important for establishing expected levels of functioning on the mental status examination. For example, the patient with a third-grade education and an inconsistent low-level work history would not be expected to perform at the level of a college graduate.

The fourth area of importance is the patient's general medical status. Many medical conditions such as endocrine diseases, chronic renal or hepatic disorders, acquired immunodeficiency syndrome (AIDS), and chronic alcohol or drug abuse adversely affect mental functioning. In some instances, particularly in elderly individuals, the use of multiple prescription and nonprescription medications can also deleteriously affect mental status.[12] When such conditions do affect mental functioning, they usually produce a confusional state, but they may mimic a dementia, depression, or other mental disorder. It is very important to diagnose these conditions early in their course because they are often completely reversible.

History Outline

The following elements in the history are particularly important in evaluating a patient with behavior change. Because such patients may not be able to provide a complete and accurate history, it is prudent to obtain the initial information from a family member or other individual who is close to the patient. Even if the patient is able to give a history, corroborative information from a second source is advisable to ensure accuracy.

1. Description of present illness
   a. Nature and date of onset
   b. Duration of illness
   c. Description of behavioral change associated with illness
2. Other relevant organic behavioral symptoms
   a. Unusual or bizarre behavior (e.g., nocturnal wandering)
   b. Evidence of poor social judgment (e.g., discarding new clothes in the trash or being verbally abusive at social gatherings without provocation); this information should be obtained from someone other than the patient

    c. Attention and concentration problems

    d. Language problems (e.g., word-finding difficulty, comprehension deficits, or tangential verbal responses)

    e. Reading, writing, or calculation difficulty (e.g., inability to balance checkbook)

    f. Memory difficulty (recent and remote)

    g. Difficulty with geographic orientation (i.e., getting lost)

3. Psychiatric symptoms

    a. Paranoia

    b. Hallucinations

    c. Delusions

    d. Depression

    e. Anxiety and agitation

    f. Other

4. Past history

    a. Previous neurologic disease or psychiatric problems

    b. Central nervous system infections

    c. Head trauma (comment on severity)

    d. Seizures

    e. Other medical disease

    f. Drug and alcohol use and abuse

    g. Use of prescription medications and over-the-counter medications

    h. Toxic exposure

5. Birth and developmental history

    a. Brain damage from birth

    b. Developmental delays

        (1) Motor

        (2) Language

        (3) Intellectual

        (4) Academic

        (5) Emotional or social

6. Educational and vocational history

    a. Highest school grade attained

    b. Adequacy as a student

    c. Vocation

        (1) Types of jobs

        (2) Frequency of job changes

        (3) Recent problems with job

7. Family history

    a. Neurologic or psychiatric disease in other family members

    b. Familial neurologic disease (e.g., Huntington's disease, Alzheimer's disease, and so on)

c. Familial predilection for a particular disease process that may involve the central nervous system (e.g. hypertension and stroke)

BEHAVIORAL OBSERVATION

The primary purpose of this section is to provide a formal framework to assist the examiner in systematically observing behavior. A careful observation of behavior is important because:

1. Several specific neurobehavioral syndromes (e.g., acute confusional state [delirium], frontal lobe syndrome, and the denial-neglect syndromes) are diagnosed primarily on the basis of their behavioral manifestations.
2. Such observations provide crucial data to aid in the differential diagnosis between organic and functional disorders.
3. A significant behavioral disturbance may dramatically interfere with subsequent formal testing (e.g., a patient in an organic confusional state will perform poorly on memory testing because of inattention). Sufficient information regarding behavior is not always available from a short period of direct observation and must also be obtained from the history provided by family members or other reliable observers.

The discussions of behavior in this chapter are primarily concerned with the identification and description of organic disease and its effects. Extensive discussions of behavior from a psychiatric viewpoint are included in all major psychiatric texts (e.g., Stevenson and Sheppe;[18] Leon, Bowden, and Faber;[11] Kaplan and Sadock[9]).

Physical Appearance

Many patients with either brain disease or functional disorders show characteristic patterns of physical appearance. Classic examples range from that of the patient with organic unilateral neglect with a total lack of attention to dress and care (e.g., shaving and washing) one side of the body, to that of the obsessive-compulsive patient who may be scrupulously dressed and groomed and unnecessarily fastidious in matters relating to cleanliness and manner. Obvious neurologic signs such as hemiplegia or chorea will not be specifically mentioned. The following aspects of appearance should be noted:

1. General appearance
   a. Descriptive data
      (1) Age
      (2) Height and weight

b. General impression of appearance
   (1) Appearance for chronologic age
   (2) Posture
   (3) Facial expression
   (4) Eye contact
2. Personal cleanliness
   a. Skin
   b. Hair
   c. Nails
   d. Teeth
   e. Beard
   f. Indications of unilateral neglect
3. Habits of dress
   a. Type of clothing
   b. Cleanliness of clothing
   c. Sloppiness in dressing
   d. Excessive fastidiousness in dressing and grooming
   e. Indications of unilateral neglect
4. Motor activity
   a. Level of general activity
      (1) Placid versus tense
      (2) Hyperkinetic versus hypokinetic
   b. Abnormal posturing
      (1) Tics
      (2) Facial grimaces
      (3) Bizarre gestures
      (4) Other involuntary movements

Mood and General Emotional Status

Mood refers to the prevailing and conscious emotional feeling. Emotional status is a general term used to indicate the patient's behavior; it may be evaluated through direct observation of the patient during the examination. Certain organic brain diseases (e.g., frontal lobe disease), as well as some psychiatric conditions, may be distinguished by rather characteristic disturbances of mood and emotional status. In addition, any disturbances of mood and emotional status may adversely affect performance on subsequent portions of the mental status examination. Accordingly, a systematic review of the following behavioral components is suggested. This is intended not to be a complete and definitive psychiatric examination but rather to provide a framework for the brief assessment of emotional status. This assessment is necessary both for the identification of organically based behavior change and for the initial differentiation of functional and organic disease. For a more comprehensive overview of the psychiatric interpretation of mood and emotional status disturbances the reader may refer to any comprehensive psychiatric text.

1. Mood
   a. Normal for the situation
   b. Sadness (hopelessness, grief, or loss)
   c. Elation (inappropriate optimism or boastfulness)
   d. Apathy and lack of concern
   e. Constancy or fluctuations in mood
   f. Inappropriate mood: expressed affect inconsistent with the content of thought
2. Emotional status
   a. Degree of cooperation with examiner
   b. Anxiety
   c. Depression
   d. Suspiciousness
   e. Anger and/or hostility
   f. Specific inappropriate emotional responses to particular situations
   g. Reality testing
      (1) Delusions (false beliefs)
      (2) Illusions (misperceptions of real stimuli)
      (3) Hallucinations
      (4) Paranoid thinking
   h. Indications of specific nonpsychotic emotional symptoms
      (1) Phobias
      (2) Chronic anxiety (generalized or specific)
      (3) Obsessive-compulsive thinking, behavior, or both
      (4) Depression
      (5) Mania
      (6) Somatic preoccupation
      (7) Dissociative symptoms
   i. Abnormalities in language or speech
      (1) Neologisms (personal formation of a new word without real meaning except to the patient)
      (2) Flight of ideas in thinking and speaking
      (3) Loose associations in thinking and speaking

Clinical Syndromes

Several distinct clinical entities are recognized primarily through behavioral observation rather than by specific cognitive testing. These syndromes primarily involve disturbances in mood, personality, and emotional reaction more than alterations in cognition. The diagnosis, therefore, is made by systematic behavioral observation.

Acute Confusional State (Delirium)

The most common of those behavioral syndromes seen in a general hospital population is the acute confusional state, or delirium. Toxic or metabolic encephalopathy is also used to describe this state. The acute confusional state has a characteristic constellation of behavioral and historic findings. The onset of symptoms is usually acute, appearing over hours or days.

Generally, the most reliable clinical feature that distinguishes the acute confusional states from other organic or functional disorders is a clouding of consciousness. Although this term may seem somewhat vague, it does accurately describe the mental state of the confused patient. Specifically, clouding of consciousness refers both to a dulling of cognitive processes and to a general impairment of alertness.[19] These patients are inattentive and produce incoherent conversations that drift from the central point; they are inconsistent and confabulatory in reporting recent events (e.g., patients may tell the examiner that they have just come back from a walk with a friend when, in fact, they have been in their hospital bed for the entire day); and they often demonstrate fluctuations in their level of consciousness. Hallucinations (often visual) and agitation are often present. Patients who are grossly confusional may be severely agitated and shout incoherently; these patients usually require restraints to prevent them from disrupting intravenous lines, urinary catheters, and other apparatus. Patients with mild confusion may appear superficially normal, but on systematic examination may demonstrate mild degrees of inattention, may be disoriented, may have difficulty holding a coherent conversation, and, on specific questioning, may admit to nocturnal hallucinations and delusions. Confusional behavior is rarely stable, and characteristically waxes and wanes throughout the day and night. At night, when environmental stimuli are reduced, the confusion and agitation often become accentuated.

The confusional state is a very important abnormal behavioral pattern to recognize because it is usually the behavioral manifestation of an acute medical problem rather than a neurologic or psychiatric condition. Toxic reactions to drugs or drug withdrawal; sepsis; metabolic imbalance; or early heart, pulmonary, or hepatic failure are common causes. Confusional behavior in the postoperative period is also extremely common. In general, elderly patients, especially those with signs of early dementia, are the most likely to develop confusional states in the aforementioned medical situations.

We have developed a delirium scale (Table 2–1) that can be particularly useful to house officers when they are first exposed to confusional patients. This scale consists of the most common clinical features of the confusional state. The examiner must make a judgment as to the presence

Table 2-1. DELIRIUM SCALE SCORESHEET*

History				
1. Speed of onset of behavior change	3	2		0
2. Fluctuation over 24 hours	3		1	0
3. Sleep-wake disturbances	3		1	0
4. Hallucinations (visual or tactile)	3			0
5. Inappropriate behavior	3	2	1	0
Clinical Features				
6. Level of consciousness	3	2	1	0
7. Psychomotor activity level	3	2	1	0
8. Incoherence and disorganization	3	2	1	0
9. Attention	3	2	1	0
10. Intelligibility of speech	3	2	1	0
11. Misinterpretation of surroundings	3	2	1	0
12. Orientation	3	2	1	0
a. Time: Year Month Date Day Season				
b. Place: State Town County Hospital Floor				
Scale: (3) 9–10, (2) 6–8, (1) 3–5, (0) 0–2				
13. Construction ability—clock drawing	3	2	1	0
Total (39 maximum)				

*3 is normal; 0 is grossly abnormal.

or absence of each feature and with many items judge the severity of the clinical feature. This scale has proved both reliable and valid in clinical use and is useful in differentiating delirium from dementia (Fig. 2–1).

Although psychiatrists or neurologists are often asked to see these patients because of their abnormal behavior or change in mental status, most patients require primary medical treatment in addition to medication for behavioral control. The confusional state may linger for many days even after appropriate medical treatment, until intracellular balance and general synaptic function are restored. During this period, tranquilizers may be used to calm the patient's agitation.

The confusional state usually results from widespread cortical and subcortical neuronal dysfunction. Cortical dysfunction causes an alteration in the content of consciousness, whereas involvement of the ascending activating system leads to the disturbances of basic arousal. With focal brain disease, confusional behavior may also be seen. This is particularly true in the first few days after an acute cerebrovascular accident or in patients who have brain tumors with associated increased intracranial pressure.

In the patient in a confusional state, further mental status testing will be affected. Inattention plus general cortical dysfunction does not allow

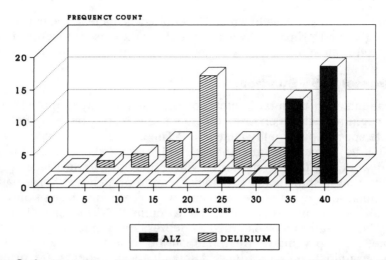

Figure 2–1. Distribution of total Delirium Scale scores of patients with Alzheimer disease versus patients with delirium. In a series of patients, it was found that delirium patients scored an average of 20 points, whereas age-matched Alzheimer disease patients scored 35.

the patient to perform adequately on memory, abstract reasoning, calculation, drawing, or writing tasks.[4] If the full test is performed while the patient is confused, a misdiagnosis of dementia can easily be inadvertently made. Because the changes in the brain are physiologic rather than structural, the patient's level of functioning should eventually return to premorbid levels; however, the confusion is often slow to clear, and definitive mental status testing to evaluate a possible underlying dementia should be postponed.

Although the acute onset of inattention, agitation, fluctuating levels of alertness, incoherent speech and train of thought, and visual hallucinations is most often due to a medical condition, the differential diagnosis must include various functional psychiatric disorders such as acute schizophrenic episode, severe anxiety or panic state, agitated depression, and mania.

The differentiation between the acute organic confusional states and acute severe functional disorders is difficult but may usually be accurately made with data provided from the patient's medical and psychiatric history, the medical examination, and some aspects of the mental status examination. Alterations in the level of consciousness are almost invariably associated with organic brain disease. Visual hallucinations are more typically seen in organic brain disease, whereas auditory hallucinations are more common in functional psychoses. Systematized delusions and organized paranoid ideation are infrequent in the patient in an acute confusional state. In any case in which the etiology is unclear, the psychiatrist, neurologist, and primary physician should work closely together to conduct a full evaluation.

Frontal Lobe Syndrome

Patients with bilateral frontal lobe disease typically do not show dramatic cognitive deficits on formal mental status testing but will often demonstrate specific personality changes.[2,13] The most common features of the frontal lobe personality are apathy, both during the examination and toward work and family; euphoria, with a tendency toward jocularity; irritability that is short lived; and social inappropriateness.[6] Some patients with frontal lobe disease are predominantly apathetic; they sit and show little interest in any aspect of their environment.[22] In such patients, the apathy is sometimes misconstrued as depression, and lengthy, expensive, and ineffective psychiatric treatment can be undertaken if a careful neurologic examination is not done. Although these patients are primarily apathetic, they may become very irritable and argumentative for short periods when sufficiently stressed.

Conversely, other patients are primarily loud, jocular, inappropriately intrusive, or socially aggressive. Because of their outgoing behavior, such patients may give the initial impression of interest and productivity. However, this emotional disinhibition and euphoria does not result in constructive activity. In general, patients with frontal damage have lost both their interest in their environment and their productive social drive. Such patients often fail to maintain job performance, normal family relations, or even personal cleanliness. Because the frontal lobes are the areas of the brain in which reason and emotion interact,[15] bilateral damage may leave the individual with apathy, unchecked emotions, and an intellect without social and emotional guidance. Other deficits that have been described in patients with frontal damage are higher-order cognitive problems, inattention, memory disorders and executive motor deficits.[13]

Behavioral features of the frontal lobe syndrome vary from patient to patient, depending partly on the locus of the lesion. Basal-orbital lesions more frequently result in disinhibited, euphoric behavior, with a lack of concern and quick irritability. In contrast, lesions involving the dorsolateral convexities tend to produce apathy, reduced drive, depressed mentation, and impaired planning.[21]

The following are two clinical examples of patients with frontal lobe syndromes:

> Mrs. L, a 58-year-old housewife, was brought to the hospital by her daughter, who reported that her mother had shown a decreased interest in caring for her house and personal needs for a year. The patient lived alone in a rural area with few neighbors. The daughter, during

an infrequent visit, had noticed a change in her mother's behavior; she showed a lack of interest in conversation and had an unkempt appearance, with a lack of concern about family affairs and total neglect of personal and household cleanliness. Neighbors had noticed that the patient had stopped attending church, did very little shopping, and no longer made social visits. On examination at hospital admission, Mrs. L was awake yet markedly apathetic. She offered no spontaneous conversation and answered all questions with only single-word responses. She walked with a slow, shuffling gait and had several episodes of incontinence. Neurodiagnostic evaluation (CT scan) demonstrated a large frontal cyst. Surgical exploration with drainage produced a marked behavior reversal. Within 2 weeks, the patient was walking well, was conversing spontaneously, and was no longer apathetic or incontinent. Mrs. L represented the primarily apathetic variation of the frontal lobe syndrome.

The following case demonstrates the disinhibition, social inappropriateness, and jocularity that may be associated with the underlying apathy in some patients with this syndrome.

Mr. N was 65 years old when brought to the hospital by his wife. Her chief complaint was that her husband's mind was deranged. The wife stated that her husband had always been a great joker but had used proper social restraint until about 4 or 5 years ago, when he had begun to show excessive candor in his remarks to friends and acquaintances. His usual outgoing personality gave way to flippancy and arrogance. His prior restraint was decreased, and he approached each social situation with an almost aggressive egotism, with much showing off and boasting.

Over the past years, he had lost regard for his personal cleanliness, bathing and shaving only at his wife's behest. His wife also reported that his memory had started to fail and that he confabulated on occasion. At one point, she had bought a new lawn mower and brought it home with the handle disassembled. She had asked him to put the handle together and to put it on the mower; he had been totally unable to do so.

Later in his course, he became quite agitated and paranoid. He wandered around the neighborhood and often told strangers fantastic tales, the last being that he "was an undercover agent for the FBI." His judgment in other matters also deteriorated. The last time he drove the car, he went through a stop sign and joked about it with his wife. These last events prompted his referral to the hospital.

Examination revealed an inattentive, restless, socially inappropriate man who was physically unkempt with uncombed hair, uncut fingernails and toenails, and messy clothes. He exhibited some paranoia, asking if his medicine (Thorazine) was some sort of poison. Several times during the examination he attempted to leave the room and was obviously agitated. His thought processes were extremely concrete, and he performed poorly on virtually all aspects of the mental status examination.

During the hospital period, he became quite upset and irritable, especially at night, and was somewhat aggressive with several nurses. The CT scan revealed frontotemporal atrophy with greatly enlarged frontal horns and widened sulci. The presumptive diagnosis in this case was Pick's disease. He died several years later, and the autopsy verified the diagnosis.

If the behavioral manifestations of the frontal lobe syndrome are present, the following neurologic diseases should be considered in the differential diagnosis: (1) tumors—subfrontal meningiomas, pituitary adenomas or primary brain tumors; (2) head trauma with frontal contusions; (3) Pick's disease; (4) general paresis; (5) communicating hydrocephalus; (6) Huntington's disease, and (7) AIDS. Any patient with extensive cortical disease (e.g., late Alzheimer's disease, multiple cortical infarcts, or traumatic or postinfectious encephalopathy) will show some of the behavior changes seen in the patient with frontal lobe disease. However, such patients also show evidence of severe cognitive dysfunction and other indications of pathologic involvement of other brain areas. Interestingly, following mild to moderate closed head injury with frontal lobe contusion, the subsequent behavioral change in certain patients is seen by family members as positive. During the past several years we have seen a number of young adult patients (usually, but not always, male) whose parents and spouses describe "improvements" in behavioral functioning in the areas of mood, reaction to environmental stress, and interactional style with others after injury and recovery from the immediate sequelae. Unfortunately, the opposite reaction—a worsening of premorbid behavioral factors—is more likely.

Disease of the frontal lobes may be difficult to evaluate clinically because of the relative absence of clear-cut cognitive changes associated with lesions of this area.[2,23] There are, however, some clinical tests that can be used to asses frontal lobe functioning. These are primarily alternating motor sequencing tasks, which have been shown by Luria[14] to be impaired in cases with extensive frontal lobe disease.

Alternating Sequences—Visual Pattern Completion

Directions: Present the patient with the visual patterns from Figure 2–2 on individual sheets of white paper. Tell the patient to reproduce the stimulus figure and then to continue the alternating sequence. If necessary, give additional elaboration of the directions to ensure that the patient

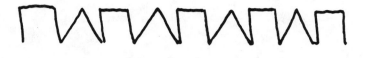

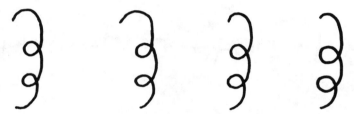

Figure 2–2. Test items for Visual Pattern Completion Test.

understands the nature of the test. Do not correct the errors or provide additional cues after the patient begins the task.

Scoring: Patients with intact motor and sensory systems should be capable of completing these sequences without error. A loss of the sequence or perseveration in the reproduction of sequences suggests a loss of the ability to move from one motor movement to another and an inability to shift sets efficiently. Examples of common errors are shown in Figure 2–3.

Alternating Motor Patterns

Directions: This test consists of a series of changes in hand position. They have been adapted from Luria[14] and are described in greater detail in that source.

1. *Fist-Palm-Side Test:* Tell the patient to hit the top of the desk repeatedly, first with a fist, then with an open palm, and then with the side of the hand. Demonstrate the task once, and then tell the patient to perform the task until told to stop. Performance for 15

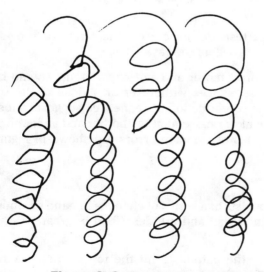

Figure 2–3. Common errors in Visual Pattern Completion Test.

to 20 seconds should suffice to assess the adequacy of these alternating movements.

2. *Fist-Ring Test:* Instruct the patient to extend his or her arm several times, first with the hand in a fist, and then with the thumb and forefinger opposed to form a ring. Demonstrate the action, and then tell the patient to perform the action. With successive extensions of the arm, the patient alternates between these two positions.

3. *Reciprocal Coordination Test:* This alternation test uses both hands. Initially the patient places both hands on the desk, one in a fist and one with the fingers extended palm down. Tell the patient to alternate the position of the two hands rapidly (simultaneously extending the fingers of one hand while making a fist with the other). Demonstrate the task.

Scoring: Normal patients should have no difficulty in easily mastering these alternating sequences after one or two attempts.[14] Accordingly, any appreciable disruption of the smooth performance of these tasks is indicative of dysfunction of the premotor areas of the cerebral cortex.

Denial and Neglect

In some patients, a brain lesion may produce a striking degree of denial of illness. The following recent case is an excellent example:

A surgeon was finishing an operation when his assistant noticed that the surgeon's left arm had suddenly become weak and his speech slurred. The surgeon was immediately put on a stretcher and was brought to the intensive care unit, where one of us saw him within minutes. The patient's arm and face were still weak, but, when asked, he replied that "it is OK." His weakness was specifically pointed out to him, and his comment was, "I really don't recognize any weakness."

This degree of denial does not seem to result from a strengthening of normal psychologic defense mechanisms but is a more basic and unusual organic behavior change. Clinically the spectrum of denial and neglect syndromes ranges from explicit denial of illness (e.g., the foregoing example), as the most severe behavioral abnormality, to a mild inability to recognize stimulation on one side of the body during bilateral simultaneous stimulation (inattention or extinction). The patient with gross denial may deny total cortical blindness (Anton's syndrome) or a severe hemiparesis (anosognosia).

In many patients with denial, the denial is more implicit than explicit. For example, when asked about the illness, the patient may not actively deny that he or she is ill but may say that the hospitalization is for tests to evaluate mild joint pain or some similar benign condition. Some patients state that they are not really in a hospital at all, but merely in a rest facility or hotel (reduplication of place or paramnesia). Such patients will often make elaborate excuses of fatigue when asked to perform with the paralyzed limb (confabulation) and on occasion will even claim that the weak arm is not theirs at all (reduplication of body parts). The surgeon mentioned earlier, for instance, claimed on the following day that he "had some arthritis" in his left arm and that was the reason for his not moving it.

Hemiplegic patients who deny weakness are a great problem in rehabilitation because they are overtly unaware of their weakness and tend to fall repeatedly. Our patient tried to walk to the bathroom on the first day after his right hemisphere stroke and fell, fracturing his left clavicle.

Some patients do not demonstrate frank denial but do have a dramatic neglect of one side of the body. Such patients may shave only one side of the face, use only one sleeve of their robe, and fail to use one side of the body even though paralysis is not present. These patients also neglect one half of the extrapersonal environment, even in the absence of a visual field defect. For example, patients may fail to respond to a visitor who approaches them from their involved side. Patients may also show neglect on drawing tasks. Examples of this type of neglect are shown in Figure 2–4.

The most subtle form of neglect is an inattention to one side of the body when both sides are simultaneously stimulated. This tendency to suppress or to extinguish the stimuli on the involved side is discussed in detail in Chapter 4.

The lesion that most frequently causes the denial and neglect syndromes is a nondominant hemisphere lesion, most frequently vascular in etiology.[5] A specific lesion locus within the nondominant hemisphere has not yet been established. Subcortical as well as cortical structures may be involved. Gross explicit denial is an uncommon behavioral finding that is most frequently seen during the acute stages after a vascular accident and is often associated with a degree of confusion. Unilateral neglect may be seen as a chronic effect of parietal lesions, predominantly in the nondominant hemisphere. The actual neuropsychologic and neurophysiologic mechanisms underlying these syndromes are not completely understood. Patients with frontal lobe disease may also show evidence of denial. For a review of this problem, see Heilman and associates,[7] Weinstein and Friedland,[24] and Weinstein and Kahn.[25]

Apathy versus Depression or Dysthymia

Apathy, lack of interest in the environment, and psychomotor slowing (psychomotor retardation) are frequently observed in patients with psychiatric depressive illness. Essentially identical symptoms, however, are also characteristic of a variety of organic brain diseases—in particular, dementia, frontal lobe lesions, and lesions in the nondominant hemisphere.

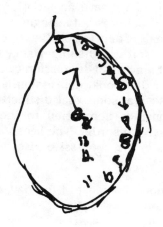

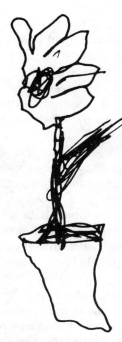

Figure 2–4. Examples of neglect on drawing test.

Many inexperienced clinicians have an unfortunate tendency to equate apathy with depression. Apathy is but a single symptom and, in isolation, never justifies the diagnosis of depression. Because of the critical difference in treatment of the two disorders, the importance of differentiating apathy of organic etiology from functional depression cannot be overemphasized.

For the purposes of this book, depression is a generic affective disorder that consists of several somewhat distinct subdisorders and many symptoms. We will consider depression to include dysthymia, major depression, and depressive disorder. The accepted DSM-III-R criteria for establishing a diagnosis of the depressive disorders are as follows:

I. Dysthymia
   A. Depressed mood for most of the day, more days than not, for at least 2 years.
   B. Presence, while depressed, of at least two of the following:
      1. Poor appetite or overeating
      2. Insomnia or hypersomnia
      3. Low energy level or fatigue
      4. Low self-esteem
      5. Poor concentration or difficulty making decisions
      6. Feelings of hopelessness
   C. During a 2-year period of the disturbance, no absence of symptoms in A for more than 2 months at a time
   D. No evidence of an unequivocal Major Depressive Episode during the first 2 years of the disturbance
   E. No occurrence of a manic episode
   F. No concomitant chronic psychotic disorder
   G. No evidence that an organic factor initiated and maintained the disturbance
II. Major Depression
   People with dysthymia often have a superimposed major depression. The primary feature of major depression is a history of one or more major depressive episodes without a history of either manic or hypomanic episodes. Some patients with major depression may have only a single episode, with full return to premorbid functioning, whereas others have recurrent depressive episodes.
   A major depressive episode is diagnosed using the following criteria:
   A. At least five of the following symptoms have been present for a 2-week period, with one of the symptoms being (1) depressed mood or (2) loss of interest or pleasure.
      1. Depressed mood most of the day and nearly every day
      2. Markedly diminished loss of almost all activities

3. Significant weight gain or loss
4. Insomnia or hypersomnia nearly every day
5. Psychomotor agitation or retardation nearly every day
6. Fatigue or loss of energy nearly every day
7. Feelings of worthlessness or excessive inappropriate guilt nearly every day
8. Diminished ability to think or concentrate, or indecisiveness, nearly every day
9. Recurrent thoughts of death or recurrent suicidal ideation

B. 1. It cannot be established that an organic factor initiated and maintained the disturbance.
   2. The disturbance is not a normal reaction to the death of a loved one.

C. There has been no recent history of delusions or hallucinations.

D. The depression is not superimposed on schizophrenia, schizophreniform disorder, delusional disorder, or psychotic disorder.

The major depression is further classified as a single episode or as recurrent, using the following criteria:

1. Major depression, single episode
   a. A single major depressive episode
   b. No history of a manic episode
2. Major depression, recurrent
   a. Two or more major depressive disorders, each separated by at least 2 months of relatively normal functioning
   b. No history of a manic episode or an unequivocal hypomanic episode

III. Depressive Disorder Not Otherwise Specified

Disorders with depressive features that do not meet the criteria for any specific mood disorder or adjustment disorder with depressed mood fall within this classification. Examples of such disorders include a major depressive disorder superimposed on a residual schizophrenia and non–stress-related depressive episodes that do not meet the criteria for a Major Depressive Disorder.

Any patient presenting with apathy of nonacute onset as an initial symptom should be carefully screened for the possible presence of a primary depressive disorder before the physician entertains a diagnosis of organic disease.

One of the most common diagnostic dilemmas is the differentiation between depression and early dementia. Both conditions are relatively common in the older population, and more importantly, they share many common features. Because of these similarities, a misdiagnosis of one for the other is all too easily made. The significance of such an error is obvious.

To tell a depressed individual that he or she is demented is a devastating error but one that is no less significant than overlooking a frontal meningioma while treating the patient for depression.

One can easily see why diagnostic confusion may occur: both conditions can present with complaints of apathy, loss of interest in work and pleasurable activities, preoccupation with minor or imagined physical complaints, difficulty concentrating, memory problems, and a general inability to keep up with the demands of everyday life. The problem is further compounded in the elderly. These patients, when depressed, do not always manifest an obviously depressive mood as dramatically as do younger patients. The elderly depressive patient also typically demonstrates fewer crying spells, less expressed sadness, less suicidal ideation (though there is no less threat of actual suicide), less expressed guilt, and less self-deprecation.[8] The elderly depressive patient may also show subtle cognitive deficits on formal mental status testing. No specific pattern of deficits is seen, and the deficits are usually mild.[3] Mild problems with concentration, memory, and arithmetic are common. There may be a paucity of details on drawings and, in general, impaired performance on any task that requires the marshaling of significant mental energy.

Because of the similarity of clinical presentation, it is not surprising that many elderly depressive patients are initially diagnosed as having a dementia.[16] The term *pseudodementia* has been applied to those patients in whom the initial diagnostic impression is of a dementia, yet on careful evaluation and follow-up, the patients' symptoms prove to be secondary to depression or another emotional disorder and improve with appropriate treatment.[10,17]

The differentiation of true early dementia from pseudodementia is not always easy. Wells[26] has tabulated the major features that he believes can help make this distinction:

	PSEUDODEMENTIA	**DEMENTIA**
Clinical course and history	1. Onset fairly well demarcated	1. Onset indistinct
	2. History short	2. History quite long before consultation
	3. Rapidly progressive	3. Early deficits that often go unnoticed
	4. History of previous psychiatric difficulty or recent life crisis	4. Uncommon occurrence of previous psychiatric problems or emotional crisis

(Continued)

	PSEUDODEMENTIA	DEMENTIA
Clinical behavior	1. Detailed, elaborate complaints of cognitive dysfunction	1. Little complaint of cognitive loss
	2. Little effort expended on examination items	2. Struggles with cognitive tasks
	3. Affective change often present	3. Usually apathetic with shallow emotions
	4. Behavior does not reflect cognitive loss	4. Behavior compatible with cognitive loss
	5. Nocturnal exacerbation rare	5. Nocturnal accentuation of dysfunction common
Examination findings	1. Frequently answers "I don't know" before even trying	1. Usually tries items
	2. Inconsistent memory loss for both recent and remote items	2. Memory loss for recent items worse than for remote items
	3. May have particular memory gaps	3. No specific memory gaps exist
	4. Generally inconsistent performance	4. Rather consistently impaired performance

In our experience, if the examiner takes sufficient time and encourages optimum performance from the patient, the depressed patient with complaints of memory loss will show normal or near-normal performance that is far better than would be expected from the nature and severity of the complaints. In some significantly depressed patients, the mental status examination seems to verify the initial impression of dementia, hence the term "pseudodementia." Because the cognitive examination actually demonstrates impairment that seems organic and is probably caused by chemical (neurotransmitter) abnormalities, the terms "depressive dementia" or "dementia of depression" have been used in preference to "pseudodementia."

The problem of pseudodementia is most commonly seen in the elderly depressed patient, but somatoform disorders, manic episodes, high levels of anxiety, and any psychotic disorder can all produce a picture of dementia on mental status examination. In these cases, it is the inattention, racing thoughts, and confused thinking that preclude adequate performance on the examination. Treating a patient with pseudodementia is rewarding because, with appropriate treatment, the patient's mental status will revert to normal, premorbid levels.

SUMMARY

Organic brain lesions may cause a multiplicity of behavioral syndromes, some of which are characteristic of specific clinical conditions. The examiner must be prepared to make a systematic evaluation of the patient's behavior and be able to recognize these major neurobehavioral syndromes. The history and behavioral observations of the patient provide essential information and serve as a framework for the interpretation of subsequently obtained data from the mental status examination.

REFERENCES

1. American Psychiatric Association: Diagnostic and Statistical Manual of Mental Disorders, ed 3 revised (DSM-III-R). American Psychiatric Association, Washington, DC, 1987.
2. Black, FW: Cognitive deficits in patients with unilateral war-related frontal lobe lesions. J Clin Psychol 32:307, 1976.
3. Caine, ED: Pseudodementia: Current concepts and future directions. Arch Gen Psychiatry 38:1359, 1981.
4. Chédru, F and Geschwind, N: Writing disturbances in acute confusional states. Neuropsychologia 10:343, 1972.
5. Critchley, M: The Parietal Lobes. Edward Arnold & Co., London, 1953.
6. Hécaen, H and Albert, ML: Disorders of mental functioning related to frontal lobe pathology. In Benson, DF and Blumer, D (eds): Psychiatric Aspects of Neurologic Disease. Grune & Stratton, New York, 1975, pp 137–149.
7. Heilman, KM, et al: Localization of lesions in neglect. In Kertesz, A (ed): Localization in Neuropsychology: Academic Press, New York, 1983, pp 471–492.
8. Janowsky, DS: Pseudodementia in the elderly: Differential diagnosis and treatment. J Clin Psychiatry 43:19, 1982.
9. Kaplan, HI and Sadock, BJ: Modern Synopsis of Comprehensive Textbook of Psychiatry. Williams & Wilkins, Baltimore, 1988.
10. Kiloh, LG: Pseudo-dementia. Acta Psychiatr Scand 37:336, 1961.
11. Leon, RL, Bowden, CL, and Faber, RA: The psychiatric interview, history, and mental status examination. In Kaplan, HI and Sadock, BJ (eds): Comprehensive Textbook of Psychiatry, ed 5. Williams & Wilkins, Baltimore, 1989, pp 449–462.
12. Levenson, AJ (ed): Neuropsychiatric Side-Effects of Drugs in the Elderly. Raven Press, New York, 1979.
13. Levin, HS, Eisenberg, HM, and Benton, AL (eds): Frontal Lobe Function and Dysfunction. Oxford University Press, New York, 1991.
14. Luria, AR: Traumatic Aphasia. Moulton & Co, The Hague, Netherlands, 1970.
15. Nauta, WJH: The problem of the frontal lobe: A reinterpretation. J Psychiatr Res 8:167, 1971.

16. Nott, PN, and Fleminger, JJ: Presenile dementia: The difficulties of early diagnosis. Acta Psychiatr Scand 51:210, 1975.
17. Post, F: Dementia, depression and pseudo-dementia. In Benson, DF and Blumer, D (eds): Psychiatric Aspects of Neurologic Disease. Grune & Stratton, New York, 1975, pp 99–120.
18. Stevenson, I and Sheppe, WM: The psychiatric examination. In Arieti, S (ed): American Handbook of Psychiatry, Vol 1. Basic Books, New York, 1974, pp 1156–1186.
19. Strub, RL: Acute confusional state. In Benson, DF and Blumer, D (eds): Psychiatric Aspects of Neurologic Disease, Vol II. Grune & Stratton, New York, 1982, pp 1–21.
20. Strub, RL: Mental disorders in brain disease. In Frederiks, JAM (ed): Handbook of Clinical Neurology, Vol 2 (46), Neurobehavioral Disorders. Elsevier Science Publishers, Amsterdam, 1985, pp 413–441.
21. Stuss, DT and Benson, DF: Frontal lobe lesions and behavior. In Kertesz, A (ed): Localization in Neuropsychology. Academic Press, New York, 1983, pp 429–454.
22. Stuss, DT and Benson, DF: Neuropsychological studies of the frontal lobes. Psychol Bull 95:3, 1984.
23. Teuber, HL: The riddle of frontal lobe function in man. In Warren, J and Alert, K (eds): The Frontal Granular Cortex and Behavior. McGraw-Hill, New York, 1964, pp 410–440.
24. Weinstein, EA and Friedland, RP: Hemi-inattention and Hemispheric Specialization. Advances in Neurology, Vol 18. Raven Press, New York, 1977.
25. Weinstein, EA and Kahn, RL: Denial of illness. Charles C Thomas, Springfield, IL, 1955.
26. Wells, CE: Pseudodementia. Am J Psychiatry 136:895, 1979.

Chapter 3

Levels of Consciousness

The initial step in administering a formal mental status examination is the determination of the patient's level of consciousness. This basic brain function determines the patient's ability to relate both to self and to the environment. Any disturbance of this elementary function will almost invariable affect the higher-level mental processes that constitute the major portion of the mental status examination. Clinically, recognizing an alteration in level of consciousness is an important indicator of brain dysfunction caused directly by primary neurologic disease or secondary to systemic illness.

The term *consciousness* is multifaceted; in testing, it is important to distinguish between the content of consciousness and basic arousal.[7] Content refers to higher cognitive and emotional functioning, whereas arousal refers to the activation of the cortex from the ascending activating system (brain stem reticular formation and the diffuse thalamic projection system). Content and arousal can vary independently, and the final level of consciousness represents a dynamic balance between cortical and ascending activating systems. This chapter deals with the clinical aspects of basic arousal.

TERMINOLOGY AND EVALUATION

There are many general terms used to describe the basic levels of consciousness, which represent points on a continuum from full alertness to deep coma. Most clinicians distinguish five principal levels: (1) alertness, (2) lethargy or somnolence, (3) obtundation, (4) stupor or semicoma, and (5) coma.

Alertness implies that the patient is awake and fully aware of normal external and internal stimuli. Barring paralysis, the patient can respond appropriately to any normal stimulus. The alert patient is able to interact in a meaningful way with the examiner. In cases of total paralysis, eye contact or eye movement may be adequate to establish this interaction. Because there are unusual comalike states in which alertness is simulated, we feel that an observation of alertness should be predicated on the clinician's impression that meaningful interpersonal interaction is taking place. Alertness per se does not imply the inherent capacity to focus attention, a topic to be discussed in detail in Chapter 4.

Lethargy is a state in which the patient is not fully alert and tends to drift off to sleep when not actively stimulated. In such patients, spontaneous movements are decreased and awareness is limited. When aroused, these patients are usually unable to pay close attention to the examiner; their eyes are open and directed toward the examiner, yet they appear dull and without animation. In conversation, the lethargic patient often loses the train of thought and wanders from topic to topic. It is difficult to validly assess memory, calculations, and abstract thinking in these patients because of their inattention and wandering thought processes. If a full mental status examination is performed in a lethargic patient, impaired performance must be interpreted with caution.

Obtundation refers to a transitional state between lethargy and stupor. The obtunded patient is difficult to arouse and, when aroused, is confusional. Usually, constant stimulation is required to elicit even marginal cooperation from the patient. Meaningful mental status testing is usually futile. The obtunded patient is, by our definition, in an acute confusional state or quiet delirium.

Stupor and semicoma are used to describe patients who respond only to persistent and vigorous stimulation. The stuporous patient does not rouse spontaneously and, when aroused by the examiner, is able only to groan or mumble and move restlessly in the bed. In such a patient, there is extensive brain dysfunction; because of the markedly reduced level of consciousness, no meaningful assessment of the content of mental functioning is possible.

Coma is traditionally applied to those patients who are completely unarousable. In coma, the patient responds neither to external stimulation nor spontaneously to internal stimulation. If coma is thus defined as a state in which no evidence of behavioral response to stimulation is present, the term can serve as an absolute end point on the scale of consciousness or arousability. Some clinicians make a distinction between light coma and deep coma. In light coma, the patient may demonstrate reflex (e.g., decorticate or decerebrate) movements but no meaningful or purposeful movements, whereas in deep coma, no motor response is seen. Stupor and coma will not be further discussed here; the interested reader is referred to Plum and Posner[7] and Fisher[2] for extensive discussions of these states.

Each of the aforementioned terms is qualitative in nature and encompasses a wide range of possible points on the continuum of consciousness. Such terms lack the objectivity and reliability that can be achieved with a less subjective assessment scheme. We suggest amending any qualitative term such as "lethargy" with a series of short statements that describe both the level of stimulus necessary to arouse the patient and the actual behavioral response elicited. First, the intensity of stimulation needed to arouse the patient should be indicated: (1) calling the patient's name in a normal conversational tone, (2) calling in a loud voice, (3) light touch on the arm, (4) vigorous shaking of the patient's shoulder, or (5) painful stimulation. Second, the patient's highest level responses should be described: (1) degree and quality of movement, (2) presence and coherence of speech, or (3) presence of eye opening and eye contact with the examiner. Finally, what the patient does on cessation of stimulation should be described.

This information can be recorded in a single statement. For example:

Patient lethargic: Name called in a normal tone of voice; patient opened eyes, pulled self part way up in bed, mumbled "why ya bothering me?" then closed eyes and went back to sleep.

Patient obtunded: Responds to loud shouting with restless movements of all extremities and brief eye opening; speech is mumbled and incoherent; when stimulation discontinued, patient returns to sleep.

Patient stuporous: Does not respond to voice but will respond to vigorous shaking of shoulder accompanied by loud calling of patient's name; patient responds with groan and aimless movement of left extremities; eyes remain closed.

These types of descriptions provide much more data on the patient's arousability and capacity for interaction than the simple terms "lethargy," "obtundation," or "stupor." It is helpful to make a chart in the progress notes so that a rapid assessment of changing levels of consciousness can be made. Table 3–1 is an example of a patient with head trauma who had a subdural hematoma. As shifts of nurses and doctors change, subtle changes in the patient's condition are easily appreciated by comparing the notes of previous observers. This system is applicable to any patient whose illness causes a decrease in the level of awareness.

Teasdale and Jennett[4,9] have demonstrated the practicality of this type of reporting system for patients with head injury. They have developed what has become known as the Glasgow Coma, or Responsiveness, Scale. It follows the conceptual scheme described earlier but has the advantage of providing a numeric score to denote the actual level of consciousness. Each level of response in the three response categories (i.e., eye opening, verbal, motor) is given a numeric value. The response is the patient's best response; it does not, however, take into account the level of stimulus required for its elicitation. The scale items and the quantitative ratings for specific responses are presented in Table 3–2.

The level of responsiveness can be assessed objectively at regular intervals and plotted as a graph. The time scale can be hourly, daily, or any selected interval. Table 3–3 is an example of such use of the scale.

ANATOMY AND CLINICAL IMPLICATIONS

The basic brain structure that is responsible for arousal is the ascending activating system. This system originates in the brain stem retic-

Table 3–1. PATIENT'S RESPONSES TO STIMULATION

	Level of Consciousness	Stimulus Necessary to Rouse Patient	Movement	Vocalization	Eye Opening	Comments
8 PM	Lethargy	Loud voice	Moved all limbs; got up on elbow	Mumbled something about being tired	Yes, with eye contact	Odor of alcohol on breath
12 AM	Lethargy	Loud voice plus gentle shaking	Moved all limbs; no attempt to rise	Incoherent mumbling	Yes, but with no sustained eye contact	Questionable Babinski's sign
4 AM	Stupor	Loud voice plus vigorous shaking	Slight movement of all extremities, but right arm not moving well	Groans	Attempted to open eyes to command	Left pupil larger than right, not as reactive; now positive Babinski's sign on right

Table 3–2. GLASGOW COMA SCALE*

Category of Response	Response	Points
Eye opening	Spontaneous	4
	To speech	3
	To pain	2
	Nil	1
Best verbal response	Oriented	5
	Confused conversation	4
	Inappropriate words	3
	Incomprehensible	2
	Nil	1
Best motor response	Obeys	6
	Localizes	5
	Withdraws	4
	Abnormal flexion (decorticate)	3
	Extends (decerebrate)	2
	Nil	1

*Adapted from Jennett and Teasdale,[4] p. 78.

ular formation and extends to the cortex via the diffuse or nonspecific thalamic projection system.[6]

A group of specialized reticular neurons in the tegmental portion of the midbrain and upper pons has the specific capacity to activate higher centers. These cells are located in a perimedian portion in the brain stem (reticular formation and locus ceruleus) and receive collateral input from most ascending and descending fiber systems. Stimulation applied to the skin of the hand, for example, will send information to the activating system as well as the sensory nuclei in the thalamus Reticular stimulation alerts widespread areas of the cortex and subcortex to the fact that an external stimulus is being applied. By this mechanism, the activating system maintains a constant, albeit fluctuating, stimulation of the higher centers. Without this steady input, the cortex cannot function efficiently; thus, the patient cannot think clearly, learn effectively, or relate meaningfully. Any damage or suppression of this system renders the patient difficult to arouse and inefficient in performance. Specific lesions such as infarcts or hemorrhages of the reticular formation lead to total disruption of arousal and, thus, to coma. Pressure on the midbrain from hippocampal or uncal herniation causes a change in the level of consciousness, which starts as lethargy but may progress to coma. Drug intoxication, disturbances in metabolic balance, and sepsis cause alterations in both reticular and cortical functioning. This leads to alterations not only in arousal, but also in the content of consciousness.

If there is damage to the extension of the brain stem reticular system in the thalamus or hypothalamus, the full picture of coma will not result. Such lesions disconnect the reticulocortical and reticulolimbic pathways

Table 3-3. GLASGOW COMA SCALE GRAPH

Patient's Response		Date	12 PM	2 PM	4 PM	6 PM	8 PM	10 PM	12 AM	
Eye opening	Spontaneous									
	To speech									
	To pain									
	None									
Best verbal response	Oriented									
	Confused									
	Inappropriate									
	Incomprehensible									
	None									
Best motor response	Obeying									
	Localizing									
	Withdraws									
	Flexing									
	Extending									
	None									
Coma Score			12	11	8	6	6	4		

and cause patients to display various interesting alterations in arousal. Because the brain stem portion of the system is intact, reticular activity innervates the nuclei of the extraocular nerves, and patients can open their eyes and look about. The cortex, however, is not sufficiently stimulated to produce voluntary movement or speech. These patients are in a comalike state.

These unusual comalike states are interesting because of the nature and degree of disturbed awareness. Some authors categorize all such cases as akinetic mutism or persistent vegetative states, whereas others prefer to separate them into many subcategories. Regardless of the terminology used, the pathology and clinical appearance of each subcategory is relatively distinct. The primary feature of these disorders is the patient's uncanny appearance of awareness. Such patients lie in bed with their eyes open and look about the room. Eye contact with others is variable. Sometimes eye movements seem random, but on other occasions, genuine interpersonal eye contact appears to take place. Other than this somewhat unnerving visual scanning, the patients remain relatively immobile and mute. It is the dichotomy between this apparent visual alertness and the lack of speech and movement that differentiates this group of patients from those in stupor or coma.

Regardless of their superficial similarity, each subgroup has its own distinct features, and it is often possible to differentiate the various states clinically. The term "akinetic mutism" seems best reserved for cases in which damage is restricted either to the midbrain or subthalamic region or to the septal region. The midbrain lesion causes a syndrome that is described as apathetic akinetic mutism. These patients are difficult to arouse but, once aroused, can move all extremities, mutter a few intelligible words, and look directly at the examiner for a few moments. They then turn away or drift back to sleep. Subtle muscle stretch reflex changes, extensor toe signs, extraocular muscle involvement, and pupillary abnormalities may be seen. This condition was originally described in a patient with a third ventricular cyst,[1] but the most common cause is occlusion of the small vessels entering the brain stem from the tip of the basilar artery.[8] This lesion interrupts the ascending activating system but not the corticospinal and corticobulbar tracts. Accordingly the patients are able to open their eyes and make some movement and sound but are unable to respond fully.

Patients with lesions that involve the septal area, anterior hypothalamus, cingulate gyri, or bilateral orbital frontal cortex are also akinetic and mute, but they appear much more alert. They are awake most of the day and have insomnia at night; their eyes remain open when awake. These patients often have violent behavioral outbursts during arousal (septal rage). Coma vigil has been used to describe these patients. This syndrome is seen with rupture of anterior communicating artery aneurysms, deep frontal lobe tumors, and anterior cingulate gyrus tumors. These patients may have increased reflexes in the legs with Babinski's signs from corticospinal tract involvement, difficulty with temperature control from anterior hypothalamic damage, and primitive reflexes (snout and grasp) from mesial frontal lobe damage. They do not have pupillary or extraocular muscle paresis. These neurologic signs, plus the more apparent alertness of these patients, frequently differentiates them clinically from apathetic akinetic mute patients.

Patients with diffuse damage to the cortical mantle from anoxia, hypoglycemia, or circulatory or metabolic embarrassment frequently survive in a state clinically similar to that of coma vigil. Their eyes are open and randomly survey the room. Brain stem reflexes are intact, but there is bilateral decortication with double hemiplegia and primitive reflexes. This condition is called the apallic state[5] because of the diffuse damage to the neocortex, or neopallium. Because of the dramatic neurologic deficit, this state should be easily distinguished from the akinetic mute states.

The term "persistent vegetative state" has been used to describe patients surviving severe head injury who are clinically similar to those in the apallic state.[3] The brain lesions are widespread at both the cortical and subcortical levels, and neurologic findings differ in each case, depending on the specific loci of the lesions. Because the term "apallic state" has never gained widespread acceptance, "persistent vegetative state" is often used for any patient with widespread brain disease and no ability to interact meaningfully with the environment.

The locked-in syndrome[7] is another comalike state that can be differentiated from the foregoing states. In this condition, a lesion (hemorrhage or infarct) in the upper pontine tegmentum interrupts all corticospinal and corticobulbar fibers at the level of the abducens and facial nuclei. Clinically, patients are unable to speak, swallow, smile, or move their limbs. In some cases, lateral gaze is also paralyzed. The entire central nervous system above the level of the lesion is intact, and these patients are literally disconnected from their motor system. These patients are "locked-in" and able to communicate only by eye movements.

Table 3–4 is a composite of the clinical features of each of these comalike states. These features plus the clinical history should enable the examiner to differentiate most of these complicated cases.

A final condition that deserves mention in this section is the state of psychogenic unresponsiveness (hysterical comalike state). This condition constitutes 1% of all patients presenting to a medical emergency room in an unresponsive state.[7] Careful examination reveals normal respiration, heart rate, and blood pressure. Muscle tone is usually decreased, but inconsistent limb tone frequently exists. All bulbar reflexes (doll's phenomenon, caloric stimulation, gag, corneal, and pupil) are intact. Muscle stretch reflexes are symmetric. Frequently, the patient will make inconsistent re-

Table 3–4. DIAGNOSTIC FEATURES OF COMALIKE STATES

Diagnosis	Level of Consciousness	Voluntary Movement	Speech	Eye Responses	Limb Tone	Reflexes
Akinetic mute (apathetic-midbrain)	Lethargy	Little and infrequent; but when sufficiently stimulated, can move *all* extremities purposefully	With stimulation, can produce normal, short phrases	Open when stimulated; usually good eye contact	Usually normal; sometimes slight increase	Can be normal; occasionally asymmetric with pathologic reflexes
Akinetic mute (coma vigil–septal)	Wakeful, with occasional outbursts; some patients somnolent	Little but purposeful; arms usually move much better than legs	Little; can occasionally produce normal phrases; also, can have outbursts of unintelligible utterances	Open during much of the day in most patients; eye contact variable	Often increased in legs	Frequently have increased leg reflexes; Babinski's signs, snout, grasp often present
Apallic state (decorticate)	Awake; no meaningful interaction with environment	No or little purposeful movement; mostly reflex or mass movements	None or occasional grunting	Open, searching, but no real eye contact	Increased in all extremities; extremities often in flexion	Increased in all extremities with pathologic reflexes
Persistent vegetative state	Awake; no or little interaction with environment	Usually little or none, depending on areas of brain damaged; mostly primitive postural reflexes	None or occasional grunts or groans; some patients produce a few words	Open, searching, but no real eye contact	Variable, usually increased; extremities often in flexion	Variable, usually increased with pathologic reflexes
Locked-in syndrome	Awake and alert; able to communicate meaningfully with examiners by eye movement	None or slight, except for eye movement	None	Open, with normal following and good eye contact; some patients have restricted lateral gaze	Increased	Increased in all extremities

sponses, such as blinking on corneal testing before the cornea is touched. Any inconsistent response gives the examiner additional confidence that he or she is not dealing with an organic coma. Psychogenic unresponsiveness should not be diagnosed too hastily; the misdiagnosis of a true coma as conversion hysteria is far more serious than the reverse.

All of the conditions discussed earlier represent disturbances of arousal caused by brain lesions or psychiatric illness. Not all alterations in levels of alertness are pathologic, however. Sleep, for instance, represents a natural fluctuation in the level of consciousness. Any degree of fatigue or sleepiness can adversely affect performance on mental status testing, even though an organic lesion is not present. Patients with brain disease will continue to have an underlying diurnal sleep-wake cycle that is superimposed on any organic decrease in alertness. It may be difficult to determine the relative effects of sleep and pathologic alterations in the level of consciousness, but the examiner must consider both factors in the evaluation. For example, the patient with head trauma who is difficult to arouse on morning rounds may only be asleep and not suffering from increasing intracranial pressure. In these critical cases, the observed level of awareness is not the only critical factor that determines the necessity for therapeutic intervention. The patient's neurologic status and overall hospital course must also be considered.

SUMMARY

Consciousness is the most rudimentary of all mental functions, and its level must be determined first in any mental status examination. Any alteration in the level of consciousness will decrease the efficiency of cortical functioning, and thereby significantly decrease the validity of the subsequent steps in the mental status examination. In the patient with diminished alertness, only the more obvious changes in higher cognitive function can be validly documented.

The arousal aspect of consciousness is controlled by the ascending activating system. Any damage to or dysfunction of this subcortical system alters alertness and thus, secondarily, affects cortical activity.

REFERENCES

1. Cairns, H, et al: Akinetic mutism with an epidermoid cyst of the third ventricle. Brain 64:273, 1941.
2. Fisher, CM: The neurological examination of the comatose patient. Acta Neurol Scand (Suppl)36:1, 1969.
3. Jennett, B and Plum, F: Persistent vegetative state after brain damage. Lancet 1:734, 1972.
4. Jennett, B and Teasdale, G: Assessment of impaired consciousness. In Jennett, B and Teasdale, G: Management of Head Injuries. FA Davis, Philadelphia, 1981, pp 77–93.
5. Kretschmer, E: Das Appalische Syndrom. Z Gesamte Neurol Psychiatr 169:576, 1940.
6. Magoun, H: The Waking Brain. Charles Thomas, Springfield, IL, 1963.

7. Plum, F and Posner, J: Diagnosis of Stupor and Coma, ed. 3. FA Davis, Philadelphia, 1982.
8. Segarra, J and Angelo, J: Anatomical determinants of behavior change. In Benton, A (ed): Behavioral Change in Cerebral Vascular Disease. Harper & Row, New York, 1970, pp 3–14.
9. Teasdale, G and Jennett, B: Assessment of coma and impaired consciousness. Lancet 2:81, 1974.

Chapter 4

Attention

After determining the level of consciousness, a careful assessment of attention is the next step in the formal mental status examination. The patient's ability to sustain attention over time must be established before the more complex functions such as memory, language, and abstract thinking are evaluated. It is of no value to ask the patient to remember the details of a story if he or she is repeatedly distracted by the nurse passing in the hall, a noise in the next room, or cars in the street. The inattentive and distractible patient cannot efficiently assimilate the information being presented during testing.

Attention refers to the patient's ability to attend to a specific stimulus without being distracted by extraneous internal or environmental stimuli.[14] This capacity for focusing on a single stimulus contrasts with the concept of alertness. Alertness is a more basic arousal process in which the awake patient can respond to any stimulus in the environment. The alert but inattentive patient will be attracted to any novel sound, movement, or event occurring in the vicinity; the attentive patient can screen out irrelevant stimuli. Attention presupposes alertness, but alertness does not necessarily imply attentiveness.

Vigilance (concentration) is the ability to sustain attention over an extended period. This capacity to concentrate is very important for performing intellectual endeavors and may be impaired in both organic and emotional disorders. The concept of inattention (distractibility) is applied to two distinct clinical situations. The first situation is when the patient is clinically inattentive or is unable to sustain sufficient attention to succeed in the simple tests of attention discussed subsequently. The second situation is when the patient has specific unilateral inattention to stimuli on the side of the body opposite a brain lesion.

EVALUATION

Observation

The most valid clinical information regarding the patient's general attentiveness may be obtained by merely observing the patient's behavior and noting any evidence of distractibility or difficulty in attending to the

41

examiner. A subjective rating scale of 0 (highly distractible) to 5 (fully attentive) is useful.

History

A patient who is having difficulty concentrating on work or other routine tasks is usually able to tell the examiner about the problem. A simple inquiry as to the patient's ability to concentrate or to sustain attention may provide revealing data.

Digit Repetition

The patient's basic level of attention can be readily assessed by using the Digit Repetition Test. Adequate performance on this task ensures that the patient is able to attend to a verbal stimulus and to sustain attention for the period of time required to repeat the digits. In patients with a significant language disorder (aphasia), this task and the "A" Random Letter Test for vigilance (see page 43) cannot be validly applied to assess attention.

Directions: Tell the patient: "I am going to say some simple numbers. Listen carefully and when I am finished, say the numbers after me." Present the digits in a normal tone of voice at a rate of one digit per second. Take care not to group digits either in pairs (e.g., 2–6, 5–9) or in sequences that could serve as an aid to repetition (e.g., in telephone number form, 376–8439). Numbers should be presented randomly without natural sequences (e.g., not 2–4–6–8). Begin with a two-number sequence, and continue until the patient fails.

TEST ITEMS

3–7	9–2
7–4–9	1–7–4
8–5–2–7	5–2–9–7
2–9–6–8–3	6–3–8–5–1
5–7–2–9–4–6	2–9–4–7–3–8
8–1–5–9–3–6–2	4–1–9–2–7–5–1
3–9–8–2–5–1–4–7	8–5–3–9–1–6–2–7
7–2–8–5–4–6–7–3–9	2–1–9–7–3–5–8–4–6

Scoring: The patient of average intelligence can accurately repeat five to seven digits without difficulty. In a nonretarded patient without obvious aphasia, inability to repeat more than five digits indicates defective attention.

Vigilance

A simple test of vigilance that can be readily administered at the bedside is the "A" Random Letter Test, consisting of a series of random letters among which a target letter appears with greater-than-random frequency. The patient is required to indicate whenever the target letter is spoken by the examiner.

Directions: Tell the patient: "I am going to read you a long series of letters. Whenever you hear the letter A, indicate by tapping the desk." Read the following letter list in a normal tone at a rate of one letter per second.

TEST ITEMS

L T P E A O A I C T D A L A A
A N I A B F S A M R Z E O A D
P A K L A U C J T O E A B A A
Z Y F M U S A H E V A A R A T

Scoring: There are currently only preliminary standardized norms for this test. The average person should complete the task without error ($\bar{x} = 0.2$); a sample of randomly selected brain-damaged patients made an average of 10 errors.[12] Examples of common organic errors are (1) failure to indicate when the target letter has been presented (omission error); (2) indication made when a nontarget letter has been presented (commission error); and (3) failure to stop tapping with the presentation of subsequent nontarget letters (perseveration error).

The Serial Sevens Subtraction Test (e.g., counting backward from 100 by sevens: 100, 93, 86 . . .) has been traditionally included in mental status examinations. Studies of performance by normal people suggest that errors on this test may reflect premorbid intellectual capability, education, calculating ability, or socioeconomic status, rather than indicating a pathologic process.[13] Excellent performance indicates adequate attention or mental control; however, failure may reflect any of a number of problems, inattention being but one. In general, this test has proved of limited validity and reliability.

Inattention

Unilateral inattention (suppression or extinction) should be tested during the routine sensory examination by using double (bilateral) simultaneous stimulation.

Directions: Double simultaneous stimulation is tested in all major sensory modalities. In tactile testing, corresponding points on both sides of the body are touched simultaneously with equal intensity. Visual testing is done by having the patient face the examiner and fix his or her gaze at a point on the examiner's face. The examiner then moves his or her fingers in right and left peripheral fields. Auditory testing is carried out by having the examiner stand behind the patient and provide a stimulus of equal intensity to each ear.

Before undertaking bilateral simultaneous stimulation, the examiner must ensure that basic sensation for each modality is intact bilaterally. If one side is inferior on unilateral testing, defects found during simultaneous testing would not necessarily reflect inattention.

Extinction is present when the patient suppresses the stimuli from one side of the body. Extinction may occur in all modalities (polymodal neglect) or may be restricted to a single modality. When extinction is elicited, the degree of inattention can be assessed by increasing the magnitude of the stimulus on the inattentive side.

When the double simultaneous stimulation includes one proximal and one distal stimulus, the distal stimulus tends to be extinguished.[3] This is particularly true when the proximal stimulus is the face and the distal one the hand. Normal adults who are less than 65 years old often extinguish the hand stimulus on the first trial, but they will usually begin to identify both stimuli after several trials. Patients with organic brain syndromes rarely recognize the hand stimulus even after as many as 10 trials. This test (Face-Hand Test)[1] is a very useful simple test for organic disease. Some normal elderly individuals will also extinguish the hand stimulus; therefore, the test must be interpreted with caution in patients older than age 65.

ANATOMY AND CLINICAL IMPLICATIONS

The basic anatomic structures responsible for maintaining an alert state are the brain stem reticular activating system and the diffuse thalamic projection system (the diencephalic extension of the reticular formation).[9]

The mechanism by which this ascending activation is focused and extraneous stimuli are screened out is less certain. Cortical and limbic stimulation can definitely influence the ascending system, so it is probable that attention results from a balance among ascending (reticulocortical) activation, ascending inhibition, and cortical (corticoreticular) modulation.[9] The importance of cortical influence in focusing attention is demonstrated in the experience of every student. Concentration while studying frequently requires conscious voluntary effort that is cortical in origin (probably widespread). The limbic system is also an integral part of the attention process; limbic input adds emotional importance to the object of attention. A child who watches a cartoon is stimulated to attention by the pleasure and excitement generated by the spectacle. The student who is studying for a test is aided in the need to concentrate by a fear of failure or a drive to succeed. These limbic influences are important and may be the critical factor that facilitates the screening out of extraneous stimuli. The principal stimulus is of greater emotional value than the incidental events in the environment, and therefore attracts greater attention.

Because attention represents a complex interaction of limbic, neocortical, and ascending activating functions, there are many areas of the brain in which damage can disrupt the ability to attend. Damage to the ascending activating system itself usually causes alterations in the level of consciousness. In such patients, alterations in attention are directly related to the more basic deficit in alertness. Inattention caused by lesions in the midbrain activating system is probably clinically rare, although a rather profound unilateral inattention has been experimentally produced in monkeys with lesions in the midbrain.[15] Inattention has also been observed clinically in patients with lesions of the thalamus,[16] the posterior internal capsule,[5] and other subcortical structures.[10]

Some of the patients who survived the encephalitis epidemic of 1918 to 1921, which was associated with von Economo's disease, were left with lesions in the ascending inhibitory portion of the reticular substance of the pons and medulla. These patients developed a behavior pattern characterized by hyperactivity and distractibility, which was called "organic driveness."[8] This state is clinically similar to that seen in some hyperactive children.

Probably the most common cause of decreased attention and vigilance in a hospital population is diffuse brain dysfunction. This dysfunction is usually caused by metabolic disturbance, drug intoxication, postsurgical states, or systemic infection. In these confusional states (deliria), all cells in the central nervous system are affected. Another common cause of inattention is extensive bilateral cortical damage of any etiology (e.g., atrophy, multiple infarcts, encephalitis, or head trauma). In patients with advanced Alzheimer's dementia, new stimuli in the vicinity may quickly draw their attention; they then become "stimulus bound" and are unable to screen out irrelevant stimuli. The cortical role in focusing and maintaining attention is very well demonstrated in these patients.

Patients with bilateral lesions of the frontal lobes or the limbic system (e.g., Korsakoff's syndrome) have a type of inattention that is characterized by indifference and perseveration. Clinically they are apathetic toward their surroundings. Test items per se have no particular interest to them. Such patients usually perform well on the digit repetition task but will not be able to complete accurately the "A" Random Letter Test. These patients will often omit an A at the end of a long sequence (e.g., U C J T O E A) because their attention has wandered. Patients with a frontal lobe lesion also have great difficulty shifting from one pattern of response to another; this deficit results in perseveration. This perseveration is commonly seen both behaviorally and on the "A" Random Letter Test. The series

E V A A R A T may be failed in the following way (italic letters indicate the patient's taps): E V *A A R A T.*

Right hemisphere lesions have a stronger effect on attention than do left-sided lesions. Denial, unilateral neglect, and extinction on double simultaneous stimulation are more frequent and prominent in patients with right hemisphere lesions.[2,6,7,11] The reason for this peculiar quality of the right hemisphere is not known. It is possible that reticulocortical or corticoreticular fibers are more dense in the right hemisphere, although there is no currently available pathologic evidence that this is true. For a thorough discussion of the theories of the inattention syndrome, see Weinstein and Friedland.[17]

Contralateral inattention to double simultaneous stimulation is seen with parietal lesions of either hemisphere. The damage to parietal tissue apparently reduces reticulocortical interaction on the damaged side, thus allowing the intact hemisphere an advantage in the stimulus rivalry.[4]

Many functional mood alterations can affect attention. Anxiety causes distractibility and difficulty concentrating; depression produces disinterest and reduced arousal. All such mood changes will hinder performance on attention tasks and will generally decrease attention.

SUMMARY

Attention results from an interplay among brain stem, limbic activity, and cortical activity that allows the patient to focus on a specific task to the exclusion of irrelevant stimuli. Both functional and organic illness can disrupt attention and cause a failure of vigilance. Assessment of attention must be done early in the mental status examination because the valid testing of many subsequent functions relies on its integrity. Inattention and distractibility can significantly impair a patient's performance on the more demanding tasks of new learning, calculating, and verbal abstraction.

REFERENCES

1. Bender, MB: Perceptual interactions. In Williams, D (ed): Modern Trends in Neurology, Vol 5. Appleton-Century-Crofts, New York, 1970, pp 1–28.
2. Bisiach, E and Vallar, G: Hemineglect in humans. In Boller, F and Grafman, J (eds); Handbook of Neuropsychology, Vol 1. Elsevier Science Publishers, Amsterdam, 1988, pp 195–222.
3. Critchley, M: The Parietal Lobes. Edward Arnold & Co., London, 1953.
4. Denny-Brown, D, Meyers, J, and Hornstein, S: The significance of perceptual rivalry resulting from parietal lesions. Brain 75:433, 1952.
5. Ferro, J and Kertesz, A: Posterior internal capsule infarction associated with neglect. Arch Neurol 41:422, 1984.
6. Gainotti, G: Emotional behavior and hemispheric side of lesion. Cortex 8:41, 1972.
7. Heilman, KM, Valenstein, E, and Watson, RT: The neglect syndrome. In Frederiks, JAM (ed): Handbook of Clinical Neurology, Vol 1(45), Clinical Neuropsychology. Elsevier Science Publishers, Amsterdam, 1985, pp 153–183.

8. Kahn, E and Cohen, L: Organic driveness: A brainstem syndrome and an experience. N Engl J Med 210:748, 1934.
9. Magoun, H: The Waking Brain. Charles C Thomas, Springfield, IL, 1963.
10. Mesulam, M-M: A cortical network for directed attention and unilateral neglect. Ann Neurol 10:309, 1981.
11. Oxbury, J, Campbell, D, and Oxbury, S: Unilateral spatial neglect and impairment of spatial analysis and perception. Brain 97:551, 1974.
12. Simpson, N, Black, FW, and Strub, RL: Memory assessment using the Strub-Black Mental Status Examination and the Wechsler Memory Scale. J Clin Psychol 42:147, 1986.
13. Smith, A: The series sevens subtraction test. Arch Neurol 17:18, 1976.
14. Umilta, C: Orienting of attention. In Boller, F and Grafman J (eds): Handbook of Neuropsychology, Vol 1. Elsevier Science Publishers, Amsterdam, 1988, pp 115–193.
15. Watson, RT, et al: Neglect after mesencephalic reticular formation lesions. Neurology 24:294, 1974.
16. Watson, RT, Valenstein, E, and Heilman, KM: Thalamic neglect. Arch Neurol 38:501, 1981.
17. Weinstein, EA and Friedland, RP (eds): Hemi-inattention and hemispheric specialization. In Advances in Neurology, Vol 18. Raven Press, New York, 1977.

Chapter 5

Language

Language is the basic tool of human communication and the basic building block of most cognitive abilities. Its integrity therefore must be established early in the course of mental status testing. If deficits are found in the language system, the assessment of cognitive factors such as verbal memory, proverb interpretation, and oral calculations becomes difficult, if not impossible.

Language disturbances are commonly seen in patients with either focal or diffuse brain disease; in fact, demonstration of a specific language disturbance is pathognomonic of brain dysfunction. Language disturbances have been well studied, and a number of distinct clinical neuroanatomic syndromes have been described. These are important to the clinician because of the relationship of specific language syndromes to neuroanatomic lesions. The ability to communicate using language is critical, and any disruption will result in a significant functional handicap for the patient.

The examiner must first develop a systematic approach to language evaluation and then become acquainted with the various classic language syndromes. Cerebral vascular accidents (strokes), brain tumors, trauma, dementia, and other lesions or diseases may all cause language disturbances. Such disturbances are not always easily characterized by a cursory examination, and a familiarity with testing and the pattern of language disruption will make the aphasic, alexic, and agraphic syndromes more understandable.

TERMINOLOGY

Dysarthria refers to a specific disorder of articulation in which basic language (grammar, comprehension, and word choice) is intact. Patients with dysarthria produce distorted speech sounds that have a variable degree of intelligibility.

Dysprosody is an interruption of speech melody. Speech inflection and rhythm are disturbed. The resulting speech production can be monotonal, halting, and can at times be mistaken for a foreign accent.

Buccofacial or oral *apraxia* is the inability to perform skilled movements of the face and speech musculature in the presence of normal comprehension, muscle strength, and coordination. When asked to show how they would blow out a match, apraxic patients may have difficulty approximating a pucker, may inhale instead of exhale, exhale vigorously without puckering their lips, or may merely say the word "blow." Any of these errors would be classified as apraxic. At times, this oral apraxia is evident only as the patient attempts to produce speech sounds; this is referred to as verbal apraxia.

Aphasia is a true language disturbance in which the patient demonstrates an impairment in the production and/or the comprehension of spoken language. The basic aphasic defect is in higher integrative language processing, although articulation and praxis errors may also be present. Aphasia usually refers to a loss of language after brain damage, but the term "developmental aphasia" is used when a child has a specific delay in language acquisition disproportionate to general cognitive development.

Alexia is the term used to describe a loss of reading ability in a previously literate person. Alexia does not refer only to a total loss of reading ability, but to any level of disturbance in reading. Alexia is not synonymous with dyslexia, which is a specific developmental learning disorder of children who have normal intelligence but who experience unusual difficulty in learning to read.

Agraphia is an acquired disturbance in writing. It refers specifically to errors of language and not to problems with the actual formation of letters or poor handwriting.

EVALUATION

The language system should be evaluated in an orderly fashion. Specific attention must be paid to spontaneous speech, comprehension, repetition, and naming. Reading and writing should be assessed after verbal language has been evaluated. A short period of systematic testing can usually identify and roughly characterize an aphasic deficit. Because the aphasic patient is always agraphic and is frequently alexic, the testing of reading and writing may be abbreviated in these cases. In the nonaphasic patient, reading and writing should be fully evaluated because alexia or agraphia, or both, may be seen in isolation. Language testing can be very comprehensive; for further information, the interested examiner is referred to the test batteries listed in Appendix 1.

Handedness

Handedness and cerebral dominance for language are closely allied; therefore, the patient's handedness should be determined before language testing. First, ask the patient whether he or she is right- or left-handed. Since many natural left-handers have been taught to write with the right hand, observation of the hand used for writing may not be an accurate reflection of natural handedness. Next, ask the patient to demonstrate which hand is used to hold a knife, throw a ball, stir coffee, and flip a coin. Also, ask the patient about any tendency to use the opposite hand for any skilled movement. In addition, a family history of left-handedness or ambidexterity is important because handedness and cerebral dominance for language are significantly influenced by heredity. The spectrum of handedness ranges from strong right-handedness to left-handedness.[20] Strong or exclusive unilateral handedness is much stronger in right-handed than in non-right-handed persons. Also, patients with a strong family history of left-handedness tend to be ambidextrous and not strongly one-handed.[25] A statement of the patient's handedness as well as the family history of handedness should be recorded.

Spontaneous Speech

The first step in language testing is to listen carefully to the patient's spontaneous speech. If the patient offers none, open-ended questions should be asked in order to elicit speech production. Listening to the patient's spontaneous speech for even a brief period may provide invaluable information that cannot be obtained during more formal aspects of the language examination. It is wise to ask the patient to discuss relatively uncomplicated issues, such as "Tell me why you are in the hospital" or "Tell me about your work." This type of general conversational question affords the patient a familiar topic and usually elicits his or her best efforts. In contrast, questions that require a mere "yes" or "no" answer will not provide sufficient speech output for meaningful evaluation. Pictures may be used to stimulate speech; however, they can restrict the range of language output because of the limitations of the specific stimulus.

Several clinical observations must be made and noted while listening to the patient's spontaneous speech. First, is speech output present? Second, is the speech dysarthric or dysprosodic? Third, is there evidence of specific aphasic errors? The most obviously abnormal output is the total lack of any speech. These patients may make some vocalizations but no meaningful linguistic utterances. This reduced output may be due to severe dysarthria, apraxia (buccofacial), or true aphasia. Next in severity is a specific aphasic disorder that is characterized by stereotyped output in which the patient repeats the same utterance in response to each question. The utterance is usually a nonsense word like "bica, bica" or "a dis, a dis, a dis." Patients with very restricted output can, however, often surprise the naive examiner by producing well-articulated curse words or short phrases when under emotional stress.

Aphasic language production is characterized by errors of grammatic structure, difficulty in word finding, and the presence of word substitutions (paraphasias). One common type of aphasic speech pattern has been classified as nonfluent.[4,19] Nonfluent output is sparse and effortful, contains primarily nouns (substantive words), is agrammatic, and contains frequent word-finding pauses. For instance, the nonfluent patient describing winter weather might say "ah, ah, chold . . . snow . . . freezing . . . ah, ah . . . cold." At the other end of the spectrum of fluency is a group of aphasic patients who produce an easily flowing speech that is remarkably empty of content and contains many abnormal words (paraphasias). Paraphasias are words that are either substitutions for the correct word (e.g., "I drove home in my pen") or contain substituted syllables (e.g., "I drove home in my lar"). The complete word substitution ("pen" for "car") is a verbal or semantic paraphasia. The syllable substitution ("lar" for "car") is a phonemic or literal paraphasia. A third variety of paraphasia is the neologistic (new word) paraphasia, which is a completely non-English word substitution (e.g., "I drove home in my strub"). Fluent aphasic speech is an easily recognizable speech pattern. The output is fluent and is characterized by normal or excessive rate of word production, often with a distinct press of speech. Content words (nouns and verbs) are lacking, and, in contradistinction to nonfluent output, small grammatic words such as articles, conjunctions, and interjections prevail. The nouns and verbs are often paraphasic. Because of the difficulty in producing nouns, word-finding pauses may interrupt the easy flow of speech. A fluent aphasic patient who was describing a picture of a man after a shipwreck said the following: "It is a . . . I can see it . . . it is near a cold and he has a . . . actually what has happened is part of a . . . the rest of it there is a man right here and he is cold being out there." Occasionally, the language of the aphasic contains so many paraphasic errors that the discourse is virtually unintelligible and impossible to follow. The term "jargon aphasia" is used for this heavily paraphasic but fluent speech.

The expressive language of many aphasics cannot be strictly classified according to fluency but, rather, is a mixture. The primary goal in the evaluation of a brain-damaged patient is to recognize that the language production is in fact aphasic. With experience, the examiner will be able to recognize accurately aphasic language and to classify the patient's language output. The classification of language output often provides important information regarding the locus of the brain lesion. Patients with nonfluent aphasia are likely to have an anterior left hemisphere lesion, whereas those with fluent aphasia usually have posterior lesions.[4] This anterior-nonfluent, posterior-fluent dichotomy holds true in about 85% of cases, but there are cases in which the reverse is true (i.e., posterior lesion with nonfluent aphasia, or an anterior lesion with fluent aphasia).[3] The classification of an aphasia does not depend on the output characteristics alone; a complete evaluation of all language functions is always indicated.

Verbal Fluency

Verbal fluency refers to the ability to produce spontaneous speech fluently without undue word-finding pauses or failures in word searching.

Normal speech requires verbal fluency in the production of responses and the formulation of spontaneous conversational speech. This ability is often impaired after brain injury, especially with anterior left hemisphere lesions, and aphasic patients will almost invariably demonstrate some impairment in fluency on formal testing. Additionally, individuals with relatively normal expressive speech and no other signs of word-finding difficulty may show subtle deficits on fluency tests. Thus, verbal fluency is a reflection of word-finding efficiency, and specifically testing this function may detect the mild language problems seen in clinically silent left hemisphere lesions or early dementias.

An overall impression of fluency is gained by listening to the patient's spontaneous speech, but subtle defects in fluency can be elicited only through specific fluency tests. Verbal fluency is typically evaluated by tabulating the number of words the patient produces within a restricted category (e.g., animal types or words beginning with a specific letter) and time limit. Two easily administered techniques are the Animal-Naming Test[24] and the FAS (controlled oral word association) test.[10]

Directions: For animal naming, instruct the patient to recall and name as many animals as possible. Any animal from the zoo, farm, jungle, water, or house is acceptable. Time the patient's performance for 60 seconds, encouraging him or her to continue whenever necessary. The score is the number of correctly produced animal names during the 60 seconds. Record the correct responses as well as any paraphasic productions.

Scoring: The normal individual should produce from 18 to 22 animal names during a 60-second period, with the expected variation being ±5 to 7.[24,41] Age is a statistically significant factor in the expected performance on this task. Normal individuals age 69 and under will produce 20 animals with a standard deviation of 4.5. This level of performance drops to 17 (±2.8) in the 70s and to 15.5 (±4.8) in the 80s. Scores less than 13 in otherwise normal patients under age 70 should raise the question of impaired verbal fluency; scores less than 10 in patients under age 80 are suggestive of a word-finding problem; in an 85-year-old, however, a score of 10 may be the lower limit of normal.

Directions: The FAS test consists of three separate, timed word-naming trials, using the letters F, A, and S, respectively. The patient is instructed to name as many words as possible (not proper names) that begin with the stipulated letter during a 60-second trial. The patient's responses, including paraphasia and repeated words, that were produced in the three 60-second trials are then recorded. Different forms of the same word count as separate responses.

Scoring: Normal people name from 36 to 60 words, with performance depending on age, intelligence, and educational level.[10] An inability to name 12 or more words per letter is indicative of reduced verbal fluency. Performance on this test should be cautiously interpreted in patients with less than 10 years of formal education.

Comprehension

Assessment of the comprehension of spoken language is the next step in the language evaluation. Comprehension must be tested in a structured fashion without reliance on the patient's ability to answer verbally. The most common error in assessing comprehension is to ask the patient to answer general or open-ended questions. Such questions require the patient to construct complex verbal answers that test the integrity of the entire language system and not verbal comprehension in isolation. Comprehension testing should require the minimum verbal response necessary for the patient to demonstrate that he or she has understood the examiner. For example, a question such as "What was the weather like in January?" does not assess language comprehension in isolation, whereas one such as "Is it snowing out today?" does.

We use two methods of testing comprehension: pointing commands and questions that can be answered with a "yes" or "no" response. Testing the patient's ability to point to single objects in the room, body parts, or articles collected from the examiner's pockets (e.g., coins, comb, pencil, key, and so forth) is an excellent way to quantify single-word comprehension. This task may be increased in complexity by requiring that the patient point to an increasing number of objects in sequence (e.g., "Point to the wall, the window, and your nose"). Increase the number of objects until the patient consistently fails. The patient of average intelligence without aphasia should succeed in pointing to four objects or more. The aphasic patient with comprehension difficulty may be able to accurately point to one or two items; therefore, it is important to continue testing until a point of consistent failure is reached. This test provides an evaluation of single-word comprehension, auditory retention, and sequence memory. For clarity, the level of performance should be described accurately on the test form. Next, a series of simple and complex questions that require only "yes" or "no" answers should be asked. For example, "Is this a hotel?" "Is it raining today?" "Do you eat breakfast before dinner?" Material may be as simple or complex as necessary. Before testing, be sure that the patient can reliably indicate "yes" and "no." Many patients will confuse these two items and be unable to speak accurately or nod appropriately. Also, it is important to ask at least six questions because correct responses can occur by chance alone 50% of the time with "yes" and "no" questions. Correct answers should alternate between "yes" to "no" randomly because of the tendency for brain-damaged patients to perseverate. It is not uncommon for a patient to answer "yes" to 10 consecutive questions without knowing the correct answer to any of them.

Many clinicians test comprehension by asking patients to carry out motor commands such as "Show me how to light a cigarette" or "Stick out your tongue." If the patient correctly carries out such commands, he or she has certainly understood them; however, many aphasic patients have significant apraxia and fail to follow the command correctly because of a problem in high-level motor integration and not because of poor verbal comprehension.

Repetition

Repetition of spoken language is linguistically and, to some extent, anatomically a distinct function. In certain types of aphasia, repetition may be either spared or involved in relative isolation. Therefore, it is clinically relevant to test this function specifically. Repetition is a complex process that can be affected by impaired auditory processing, disturbed speech production, or disconnection between receptive and expressive language functions.

Testing should be done with material of ascending difficulty. Begin with single, monosyllabic words and proceed to complex sentences. The following list of items provides a suitable range of difficulty. The patient should be asked to repeat the word or sentence verbatim after the examiner.

1. Ball.
2. Help.
3. Airplane.
4. Hospital.
5. Mississippi River.
6. The little boy went home.
7. We all went over there together.
8. The old car wouldn't start on Tuesday morning.
9. The fat short boy dropped the china vase.
10. Each fight readied the boxer for the championship bout.

The examiner must listen for paraphasias, grammatic errors, omissions, and additions. Normal people and nonaphasic brain-damaged patients can accurately repeat sentences of 19 syllables.[38] Performance is related to intelligence and educational level, but errorless performance is expected on these specific items.

Naming and Word Finding

The ability to name objects is one of the earliest acquired and most basic language functions. It is almost invariably disturbed in all types of aphasias.[24] Word-finding difficulty is closely related to impaired naming ability (anomia) and refers to a reduced ability to retrieve the nouns and verbs used in spontaneous speech. Specific word-finding problems can be detected by listening to the aphasic patient's spontaneous speech. Asking the patient to describe a picture that contains objects and actions will dramatize the word-finding defect. Anomia may also be objectively tested with a confrontation naming test. In this task, the examiner points to a variety of objects or pictures of objects and asks the patient to name them. The examiner should select from 10 to 20 items. Several categories of objects should be used (colors, body parts, room objects, articles of clothing, and parts of objects). Various categories are chosen because some aphasic patients have a curious inability to name objects in a specific category while maintaining adequate ability to name objects in other categories. Because the disruption of naming has varying degrees of severity, it is important to use uncommon (low frequency of usage) items as well as common (high frequency of usage) items. For example, "nose," "arm," and "floor" are common, high-frequency words, whereas "watch stem and crystal," "shin," and "coat lapel" are uncommon, low-frequency words. Many aphasic patients will be able to name common objects quickly and accurately, only to show great hesitancy, paraphasia, and circumlocution with uncommon objects. Some patients obviously recognize the object and are able to demonstrate and describe its use but cannot name it. For example, a patient shown a door key responded with "Oh, you know . . . the thing used to get in the . . . you turn it to get in."

The 20 items in Table 5–1, listed in ascending order of difficulty, are suggested for evaluating naming ability. Normal individuals will know all items except the parts of objects; on this set of five words the average score is 4.5 (± 0.8). The examiner should note that the names for parts of objects are low-frequency words and will be frequently misnamed or not named by most aphasic patients and patients with early dementia.

Table 5–1. OBJECTS FOR CONFRONTATION NAMING IN ASCENDING ORDER OF DIFFICULTY BY CATEGORY

Colors	*Body Parts*
Red	Eye
Blue	Leg
Yellow	Teeth
Pink	Thumb
Purple	Knuckles
Clothing and Room Objects	*Parts of Objects*
Door	Watch stem (winder)
Watch	Coat lapel
Shoe	Watch crystal (lens)
Shirt	Sole of shoe
Ceiling	Buckle of belt

With experience, each examiner will develop a personal repertoire of items tailored to his or her own office and patient population.

Reading

Reading ability is one of the few aspects of mental status testing that is directly related to educational experience. It is important, therefore, to determine the patient's educational background before testing reading. Demonstrating an alexia (reading deficit) in a patient only to discover that he or she has had but 3 years of formal education is merely documenting the patient's illiteracy.

Both reading comprehension and reading aloud should be tested. Both are usually defective in the same patient, but either can be disturbed in isolation. If the patient is not aphasic, screen for alexia by having the patient read a paragraph from a newspaper or magazine. To test reading in the aphasic patient, begin with reading short single words, then phrases, sentences, and finally paragraphs. First, have the patient read the item aloud, and then have him or her indicate comprehension by pointing to the object or saying or nodding "yes" or "no." For example, if the patient read the sentence "The boy or girl walked in the snow," the examiner could ask, "Did the boy go alone?" or "Was it raining when the boy and girl went for a walk?"

The examiner should note any syllable or word substitutions (paralexic errors), omitted words, and defects in comprehension. Occasionally, patients have visual field defects or problems in ocular motility. In such cases, the examiner must assist the patient stay on the written line and ensure that the patient completes one line before starting another. Using careful observation and examination, the examiner can readily separate the patients with true alexia from those having problems with the mechanics of reading.

Writing

Writing must be tested in the same careful way as that used to test reading. If the patient shows evidence of aphasia, he or she will undoubtedly have an agraphia. First, have the patient write letters and numbers to dictation. Second, ask the patient to write the names of common objects or body parts. Third, if the patient can successfully write single words, ask him or her to write a short sentence describing the weather, his or her job, or a picture from a magazine. Asking the patient to write his or her name is not always meaningful because name writing may be preserved even in the presence of gross agraphia. In the literate, nonaphasic patient, the examination can begin with this sentence-writing task. Writing to dictation is a somewhat different task that can also be tested if time allows.

The aphasic patient who is unable to write spontaneously may show residual writing ability when asked to write to dictation.

Agraphia is diagnosed when basic language errors, gross spelling errors, or paragraphias (word or syllable substitutions) are present.

Writing can often show a misalignment, in which the written line slants upward or downward. This misalignment is an error in the mechanics of writing but is not an agraphia per se.

Spelling

Spelling is a complex, little studied, higher-language function that is strongly associated with educational experience. For practical purposes, spelling can be evaluated by asking the patient to spell dictated words. Gross errors in spelling can be detected in bedside testing; if it is important to establish an actual level of competence, standardized achievement tests should be used (see Appendix 1).

CLINICAL IMPLICATIONS

Cerebral Dominance

Approximately 90% of the population is considered definitely right-handed. Of this 90%, more than 99% are strongly left hemisphere–dominant for language.[6] Because of this strong language dominance in right-handed individuals, left hemisphere lesions will frequently cause aphasia, whereas right hemisphere lesions rarely result in such deficits (i.e., a crossed aphasia).[42] Left-handed individuals (non–right-handers) have a far different pattern of cerebral dominance for language. In 80% some degree of language representation exists in both hemispheres.[22] In individuals with a strong family history of left-handedness (non–right-handedness or sinistrality), this mixed dominance tends to be more prominent. Strongly left-handed individuals with no history of familial sinistrality tend to have the strongest left hemisphere dominance for language of all left-handed individuals. Accordingly, damage to either hemisphere in a left-handed patient will result in aphasia in 80% of all cases. The aphasia will be less severe than that resulting from a similar lesion in the left hemisphere of a right-handed patient. Knowing the patient's cerebral dominance for language is important for localizing lesions and for deciding the risk to language of neurosurgical procedures. In cases in which documentation of hemispheric dominance for language is critical (e.g., left-handed patient with a right middle cerebral artery aneurysm), an intracarotid Amytal injection (Wada test) at the time of angiography can often establish dominance.[40]

Aphasia Syndromes

The impairment of language secondary to brain damage is not a unitary process; all components of language can show variable disruption. The extensive study of right-handed aphasic patients has resulted in a generally accepted schema of cortical regionalization of language. Because there are some overlapping features among aphasic patients who demonstrate a picture of mixed aphasia, some aphasiologists do not believe that this traditional neurologic classification system is suitable for neurolinguistic research.[12] However, this classification system follows the classic anatomic pattern, is easy for the student to understand, and is useful to the clinician for localizing lesions.

The posterior language area (area 1, Fig. 5–1) is the cortical area primarily concerned with the comprehension of spoken language. This area has traditionally been referred to as Wernicke's area, although the exact boundaries of the region have not been agreed on.[8] The anterior language area (area 2, Fig. 5–1) subsumes the functions of language production. Brodmann's area 44 within the anterior language area is the classic Broca's area. Recent positron emission tomography (PET) studies of glucose metabolism have supported this regional specialization in aphasic patients but have demonstrated that almost all aphasics, irrespective of clinical characteristics, have evidence of hypometabolism in the temporal region on the left.[29] Such studies demonstrate that the language system is

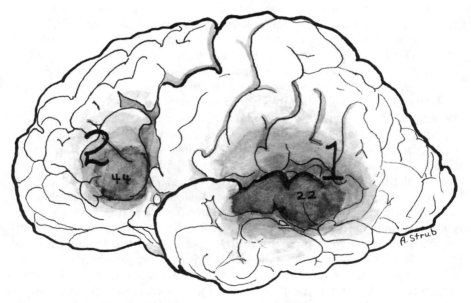

Figure 5–1. Anterior and posterior language areas.

quite complex physioanatomically and is not simply a collection of cortical centers that act independently.

Traditionally, patients with damage in the posterior speech area are called "receptive aphasics" because of their primary difficulty in understanding spoken language. Patients with lesions in the anterior area are called "expressive aphasics" because of their primary difficulty in producing language. The problem in using the term expressive aphasia is that all aphasics have some type of abnormal language expression. For this reason, we prefer to use the classification system described hereafter rather than the expressive-receptive dichotomy.

The clinical features of a patient's aphasia change dramatically over time. The acute destructive lesion causes maximal language disruption and is often associated with considerable disorientation and confusion. In the first several weeks, recovery is rapid and the aphasic picture constantly changes. After approximately 3 to 4 weeks, the aphasic pattern is more stable and may be fully assessed. The final prognosis of language recovery, however, cannot be given at that time because the reorganization and recovery process can continue for months or even years.

Global Aphasia

Global aphasia, the most common and severe form of aphasia, is characterized by spontaneous speech that is either absent or reduced to a few stereotyped words or sounds (e.g., "ba, ba, ba" or "dis, a dis, a dis"). Comprehension is absent or reduced to only recognition of the patient's name or a few selected words. Performance on repetition is at the same level as spontaneous speech. Reading and writing are likewise severely impaired. Global aphasia is caused by a large lesion that damages most or all of the combined language areas 1 and 2 (anterior and posterior shaded areas). The most common lesion is an occlusion of the internal carotid artery or the middle cerebral artery at its origin. Unfortunately the prognosis for language recovery in these patients is poor. Global aphasia is almost always associated with hemiplegia. Because of these combined deficits, such patients have a severe chronic disability.

Broca's Aphasia

This classic syndrome has as its hallmark nonfluent, dysarthric, effortful speech. The patient utters mostly nouns and verbs (high-content words), with a paucity of grammatic fillers. The characteristic speech has been called agrammatic or telegraphic. For example, one Broca's aphasic patient described a picture of a boy on a stool stealing cookies while his mother is washing dishes and letting the sink run over[24] in the following manner: "Boy . . . ah girl steal cookie . . . stool falling . . . water spilling . . . dishes." Repetition and reading aloud are as severely impaired in these patients as is their spontaneous speech. Auditory and reading comprehension are surprisingly intact, although the comprehension of complex grammatic phrases (e.g., "Do you eat lunch before breakfast?") is often impaired. Naming may show paraphasic responses.

This characteristic nonfluent aphasic syndrome results from a lesion in the anterior speech area (area 2, Fig. 5-1). The lesion causing Broca's aphasia includes more than area 44 alone. Lesions restricted exclusively to area 44 result in only transient dysarthria or dysprosody.[30] Auditory and visual (reading) comprehension are intact because parietal and temporal lobes are not damaged. Patients with Broca's aphasia usually have right hemiplegia.

These patients often undergo an interesting and significant emotional change, characterized by frustration, agitation, and depression.[5] Whether this emotional change is a functional reaction to the loss of speech or a specific organic change associated with left frontal lobe damage is not yet known.[37]

The prognosis for language recovery in patients with Broca's aphasia is generally more favorable than in those with global aphasia. Because of relatively intact comprehension, these patients adjust better to life situations.

Wernicke's Aphasia

Wernicke's aphasia can be considered the linguistic opposite of Broca's aphasia. The patient with Wernicke's aphasia has fluent, effortless, well-articulated speech. The output, however, contains many paraphasias and is often devoid of substantive words. There is often a great press to speak. The following is an example of speech in Wernicke's aphasia. The patient was a ferry boat captain with a left temporal lobe brain tumor. In describing his previous work, the patient said, "Yea, I walked on the . . . always over . . . then pull it in . . . tie the . . . ah, ah over and back over wellendy catch it. . . . " The spontaneous speech can range from comprehensive sentences with occasional paraphasic errors to totally incomprehensible jargon in which most words are paraphasias and the output is empty and devoid of content.

The essential feature of Wernicke's aphasia is a severe disturbance of auditory comprehension. Because the comprehension defect is so marked, the patient answers questions inappropriately and is completely unaware that the answers are often total nonsense. Repetition is severely impaired because of a severe auditory processing defect. Naming is grossly paraphasic. Reading and writing are also markedly impaired.

The lesion that causes Wernicke's aphasia is in the posterior language area (area 1, Fig. 5-1). The more severe the defect in auditory comprehension, the more likely it is that the lesion involves the posterior portion of the superior temporal gyrus. If single-word comprehension is good, yet comprehension of complex material is impaired, the lesion is more likely to involve the parietal lobe rather than the superior temporal lobe.[24] Because the damage is restricted to parietal and temporal lobes in most patients, the classic Wernicke's aphasic patient does not have hemiplegia.

The Wernicke's aphasic patient is often initially considered to be psychotic rather than aphasic by family and medical personnel alike. This confusion arises because the patient usually does not have a hemiplegia and produces inappropriate, but often reasonably well formed, sentences. The gross comprehension deficit may not be appreciated, and the inappropriate answers to the examiner's questions are judged to be due to a basic thought disorder rather than a language disorder. The patient's brain damage is overlooked because of the absence of neurologic findings such as hemiparesis, sensory loss, or altered level of consciousness. These patients can often develop unusual patterns of behavior. They are frequently totally unaware of their problem and talk endlessly without the slightest appreciation of their language deficit. This indifference may approach the point of euphoria. Other patients, however, develop a pronounced paranoid attitude accompanied by combative behavior.[5] This behavioral change may become chronic and require use of major psychotropic medication or treatment in a long-term psychiatric facility.

Patients with severe comprehension deficits do not have a good prognosis for language recovery, even with intensive language therapy. Milder Wernicke's aphasia may evolve into conduction or anomic aphasia—conditions in which auditory comprehension is adequate, but output contains paraphasias and word-finding pauses.

Conduction Aphasia

The hallmark of conduction aphasia is a disproportionate deficit in repetition. This syndrome is characterized by fluent, yet halting, speech with word-finding pauses and literal paraphasias. Comprehension is good, naming is mildly disturbed, and repetition is severely defective. This syndrome demonstrates that repetition and propositional speech (everyday language used to describe events or thoughts) are distinct psycholinguistic processes that can be selectively impaired by focal brain lesions. In conduction aphasia, reading is quite good, but writing shows errors in spelling, word choice, and syntax.

Two lesions are known to cause this type of aphasia. The first is usually reported to involve the supramarginal gyrus and arcuate fasciculus, a long fiber tract between the anterior and posterior areas (Fig. 5–2). The second lesion damages the insula, contiguous auditory cortex, and underlying white matter. This lesion spares the arcuate fasciculus, which arches higher into the parietal operculum.[16] This entity represents one of the clinical disconnection syndromes[18] because it literally disconnects the auditory sensory cortex from the motor speech cortex.

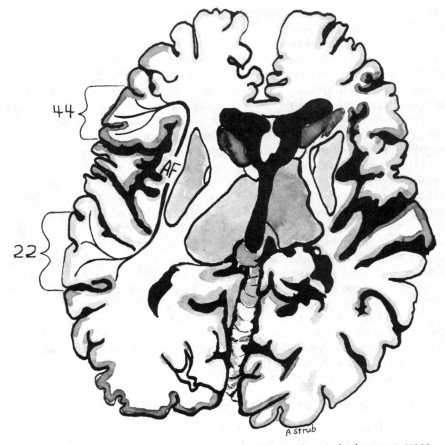

Figure 5–2. Arctuate fasciculus (AF) and anterior and posterior language areas.

Transcortical Aphasias

The linguistic opposite of conduction aphasia is transcortical aphasia. The transcortical aphasias are characterized by intact repetition of spoken language but disruption of other language functions. Some patients will have difficulty producing language but have adequate comprehension; others will produce fluent speech but have poor comprehension.

The patient with transcortical motor aphasia is able to repeat, comprehend, and read well but has the restricted spontaneous speech of the patient with Broca's aphasia. In contrast, the patient with transcortical sensory aphasia repeats well but does not comprehend what he or she hears or repeats. Spontaneous speech and naming are fluent but paraphasic, as in Wernicke's aphasia. Occasionally a patient may have a combination of transcortical motor and sensory aphasias. These patients are able to repeat long sentences, even in a foreign language, with remarkable accuracy. Repetition is very easy to initiate in these patients, even inadvertently, because they have a tendency to be echolalic (to repeat everything said within the range of their hearing).

The lesions that cause transcortical aphasia are extensive, crescent-shaped infarcts within the border zones between major cerebral vessels (e.g., within the frontal lobe between the territories of the anterior and middle cerebral arteries). Transcortical motor aphasia is seen with an anterior border zone lesion that resembles a reversed C (Fig. 5–3). These lesions spare the superior temporal and inferior frontal cortex (areas 22 and 44 and their immediate environs) and the parietal perisylvian cortex. This spared perisylvian cortex is all that is required for complete and accurate language repetition. When this region is the only language area spared by combined borderzone infarcts, the resulting language deficit (echolalia) has been called the isolation of speech syndrome.[21] The most common causes of the transcortical aphasias are (1) anoxia secondary to decreased cerebral circulation, as seen in cardiac arrest; (2) occlusion or significant stenosis of the carotid artery; (3) anoxia due to carbon monoxide poisoning; and (4) dementia.[9,36]

Recovery from transcortical sensory aphasia is relatively good, but few data are available regarding the prognosis in the motor or mixed transcortical aphasias.

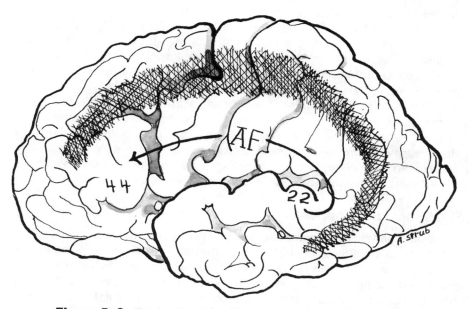

Figure 5–3. Border-zone infarct that produces transcortical aphasia.

Anomic Aphasia ·

There are aphasic patients whose only language defects are word-finding difficulty and an inability to name objects on confrontation. This condition has been labeled anomic, nominal, or amnestic aphasia. Spontaneous speech is usually fluent and grammatically rich but contains many word-finding pauses and paraphasias of specific object names. Auditory comprehension is very good, except when the patient is asked to point to a series of specific objects. This comprehension defect is a result of two-way dissociation of naming: the patient cannot name objects and frequently has difficulty recognizing object names when offered in examination. Repetition is good, with the exception of sentences that contain many nouns. Reading and writing may be impaired in specific patients; the degree of alexia and agraphia depends entirely on the location of the lesion that is responsible for the aphasia.

Lesions in many parts of the dominant hemisphere can cause anomic aphasia; thus, the localizing significance of this type of aphasia is limited. Neurosurgical mapping studies of naming have demonstrated multiple sites where naming can be interrupted with a low-level electric current.[34] The sites differed widely among patients, and the only area that produced naming problems in more than 50% of the patients was the postero-inferior frontal cortex. The most severe anomic aphasia, however, is noted in patients with temporal lobe lesions involving the second and third temporal gyri. This area cannot be considered an actual "word dictionary" but includes important pathways from the occipital lobe to the limbic system that are critical for object naming.[18] Lesions in the parietotemporal area also result in rather severe anomia. Patients with these lesions also have significant alexia with agraphia. Accordingly, the combined syndrome of alexia and agraphia with anomic aphasis will localize a lesion to the left parietotemporal area.

Anomias may be so mild that they are scarcely detectable in normal conversation or so severe that spontaneous output is nonfluent and empty of meaningful content. The prognosis for language recovery depends on the severity of the initial defect. Because language output is relatively spared and comprehension is reasonably intact, such patients make better life adjustments than other, more severely affected aphasic patients.

Subcortical Aphasia

Some patients with vascular lesions (either hemorrhage or infarct) of the thalamus, putamen-caudate, or internal capsule will demonstrate aphasic symptoms. They are dysarthric and often run words together. They have mild anomia and comprehension deficits, yet have excellent repetition.[15,31] Anterior lesions tend to produce speech-production problems; posterior lesions result in comprehension difficulty.[32]

The mechanisms by which these subcortical lesions produce aphasia are not clear. In some cases, the disorder seems more a motor-speech problem; in others, a true aphasia or language disturbance is present.[26] Because the cortex is thought to be the repository of language engrams, it is most likely that the subcortical damage alters the input to and the function of the overlying cortex. In one study of glucose uptake in subcortical aphasic patients, Metter and associates[28] demonstrated a definite decrease in cortical metabolism in addition to the expected decreased metabolism of the subcortical structures.

Aphasia in Left-Handed Individuals (Non–Right-Handers)

Owing to their mixed dominance, the left-handed individual is likely to become aphasic secondary to a lesion in either hemisphere. The resultant aphasia is usually milder and shows greater recovery than does an aphasia due to a similar lesion in a right-handed patient. In 35% to 40% of the cases, the aphasia cannot be classified within the traditional scheme. Wernicke's aphasia or the agrammatism of Broca's aphasia is rarely seen. Decreased verbal fluency and dysarthria are common, but comprehension is usually relatively intact. Repetition is relatively spared. Naming and reading are defective when the patient's lesion is in the left hemisphere.[11,23]

Language in Alzheimer's Disease

A progressive deterioration in language facility is observed in atrophic (cortical) dementia. In the earliest stage, the patient's conversation wanders in a circumlocutory fashion and can be difficult to follow. The content of conversational speech is simplified and reflects the general decrease in intellectual ability. Word-finding pauses may be present and verbal fluency is reduced. As the disease progresses, word-finding difficulty becomes prominent and paraphasic substitutions are seen. Spontaneous speech lacks relevance and may be tangential. Intrusions of words or phrases from earlier parts of a conversation may appear at inappropriate times. Comprehension is also decreased. Naming is reduced and may be paraphasic. Repetition, however, is preserved quite late in the course of the dementia.

In the late stages of the disease, there is little spontaneous speech or comprehension. Echolalia is often seen. In the final decorticate state, the patients become mute.[1,13]

Progressive Aphasia

An interesting progressive language disorder is caused by relatively restricted left frontotemporal degeneration. Such patients generally show a slowly progressive nonfluent aphasia and apraxia, with good preservation of comprehension and other cognitive functions for many years. Many eventually become demented in the late stages of their illness. Pathologically these cases are mixed: some show findings of Alzheimer's disease; some, Pick's disease; and some, Creutzfeldt-Jakob spongiform encephalopathy and other degenerative disorders.[7,27]

Pure Word Deafness

Pure word deafness is a rare syndrome in which patients do not have aphasic speech, agraphia, or alexia yet have a total lack of comprehension of verbal language. Hearing is intact, and they recognize nonlanguage sounds (auditory gnosis).

The lesion that produces this condition is located in the posterior language area and is usually bilateral. The deep lesion in the temporal lobe disconnects auditory input from the auditory cortex.[2]

Articulation Disturbances

Dysarthria

Pure dysarthrias are caused by a disruption in any of the inputs to the muscles of articulation: the cortex, as in Broca's aphasia; the basal ganglia, as in parkinsonism or cerebral palsy; bilateral striatal or pontine lesions, as in pseudobulbar palsy; or the bulbar neurons, as in amyotrophic lateral sclerosis. The patient with pure dysarthria can communicate normally using reading and writing.

Apraxia

Buccofacial apraxia may be caused by various lesions between the supramarginal gyrus and the frontal lobe in the dominant hemisphere. Lesions in these areas appear to interrupt the motor planning necessary for the complex movements of normal speech. Many aphasic patients, particularly those with Broca's or conduction aphasia, have considerable apraxia of facial movement. Some patients with language output resembling Broca's aphasia may, in fact, have pure buccofacial apraxia. The difficulty in separating the aphasic and apraxic components of speech in some patients has resulted in some speech pathologists considering Broca's aphasia as merely a motor-speech disorder and not a true aphasia. Broca's aphasia can be seen, however, in the absence of any buccofacial apraxia. Therefore, careful examination of each patient is important to separate the apraxic and aphasic components.

Dysfluency

Dysfluency (stuttering or stammering) is another speech-production problem. Not an aphasia, apraxia, or dysarthria, it is a common speech disorder whose exact etiology is not known. Both organic and functional explanations have been advanced but not proved. Dysfluency may be acquired secondary to a brain lesion or may be developmental in nature.

Alexia

There are several distinct syndromes in which reading ability is impaired by acquired brain lesions. The classic syndrome of pure alexia without agraphia[17,18] is caused by a left posterior cerebral artery occlusion in a right-handed individual. The resulting cerebral infarct damages the posterior portion of the corpus callosum as well as the left occipital lobe. Because the left visual cortex is damaged, all visual information enters only the right hemisphere. The right visual cortex perceives the written material but is unable to transmit it to the left hemisphere because of the

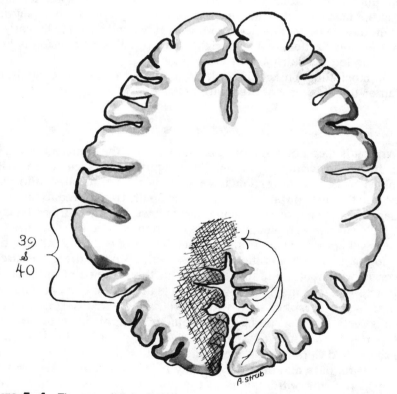

Figure 5–4. The cross-hatched area represents infarction of the left visual cortex and the posterior portion of the corpus callosum. The visual information from the right visual cortex *(arrow)* is unable to reach the left inferior parietal lobule (39 and 40) because of the callosal lesion.

callosal lesion (Fig. 5-4). The inferior parietal lobule in the dominant hemisphere (primarily area 39, the angular gyrus) is the association cortex that combines the visual and auditory information necessary for reading and writing. In alexia without agraphia, the inferior parietal lobule is disconnected from all visual input. Because the lobule and its connections within the language area are intact, the patient can write normally. One of the dramatic aspects of this syndrome is the patients' ability to write lengthy, meaningful messages, only to be unable to read his or her own writing. These patients are able to understand words spelled aloud. Interestingly, most patients with this syndrome can name objects and discuss visual events that are occurring in their environment. This type of visual information must cross to the left hemisphere by some pathway other than the damaged posterior corpus callosum.

A second distinct type of alexia results from damage to the inferior parietal lobule itself (angular gyrus and environs). This lesion renders the patient unable to read or write. This syndrome is classically called alexia with agraphia. These patients are not appreciably aphasic but may have a certain degree of anomia. Recognition of this syndrome is clinically important for localization, as in the right-handed patient the lesion is invariably in the left inferior parietal area.

The most common acquired alexia is neither of the pure syndromes but rather the alexia associated with aphasia.

Agraphia

Writing is a complex motor task that involves the translation of a language item into written symbols. The linguistic message to be written originates in the posterior language area, is then translated into visual symbols in the inferior parietal area, and is finally transferred to the frontal language area for motor processing. Lesions within any of these language areas will cause an agraphia. With the exception of patients with pure word deafness, all aphasic patients show some degree of agraphia. Although the most common agraphia is the form seen with aphasia, there are circumstances in which agraphia may be seen in the absence of aphasia. Two syndromes are seen in patients with damage in the dominant parietal lobe: the first is the agraphia seen with alexia, which was described in the previous section; the second is a syndrome of agraphia in association with other parietal lobe signs (dyscalculia, right-left disorientation, and finger agnosia), called Gerstmann's syndrome (discussed in detail in Chapter 9).

One rare, pure agraphia occurs only in the left hand. This syndrome is seen in patients with lesions of the anterior corpus callosum. These patients are agraphic with the left hand only, because the right motor cortex is disconnected from the language areas of the left hemisphere. Writing with the right hand is normal because of the intact connections of

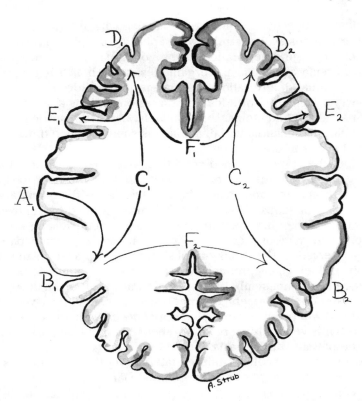

Figure 5–5. The written message originates in the posterior language area of the dominant hemisphere (B_1). The message is transferred via the arcuate fasciculus (C_1) to the premotor area in the same hemisphere (D_1). Motor patterns are transferred to the motor strip (E_1) for innervation of the right hand. The message must cross via the anterior corpus callosum (F_1) to the right motor system (D_2, E_2) for innervation of the left hand. F_2 is not a significant pathway for transferring the written message to the right motor area.

the left motor cortex and the language areas. Figure 5–5 demonstrates the normal pathways required for writing. The callosal lesion (F_1) appears to interrupt the language message going to the right hemisphere.

There are also single case reports in which isolated pure agraphia has been seen as a result of superior parietal lesions.[39]

Psychotic Language
(Bizarre Language Output)

Rambling, disjointed, neologistic language can be seen in patients with severe psychosis (especially schizophrenia), advanced organic dementia, delirium, and fluent jargon aphasia. Differentiation among these conditions on the basis of spontaneous speech alone may be difficult. Historical data are invaluable: an acute onset of gross language disturbance in the elderly favors the diagnosis of a stroke with aphasia or delirium; a prolonged history of language deterioration in the young patient favors a diagnosis of schizophrenia or an unusual organic lesion such as a left hemisphere glioma; a gradual deterioration of language in the older patient suggests a diagnosis of dementia or a focal brain lesion such as a left hemisphere tumor or subdural hematoma. Unfortunately, detailed historic information is often unavailable, and a tentative diagnosis must at such times be based on mental status findings alone.

Each of the aforementioned conditions has certain features that help to distinguish it from the others. Systematized paranoid delusions may be seen in both aphasia and dementia; however, such delusions are much more common in schizophrenia. Neologisms produced by schizophrenic patients tend to be infrequent in number, but, when present, are usually consistent and symbolic (e.g., one paranoid schizophrenic patient repeatedly referred to the "frinky-franks" that were placed in the walls to watch him). Neologisms produced by aphasic patients tend to be random, very frequent, and nonsymbolic (e.g., "The walret is the you know, wimbit, lep, olla other one"). Demented patients will frequently have word-finding difficulty and will produce circumlocutory speech with some paraphasias. Their speech is generally more comprehensible and less paraphasic than that of the patient with aphasia.

Because it is difficult to differentiate among these conditions by listening to spontaneous speech alone, complete language testing is essential. Careful comprehension testing reveals that jargon aphasic patients are unable to understand even very simple commands. Demented, delirious, or schizophrenic patients will have adequate comprehension, but they may be difficult to evaluate because of a lack of cooperation. Testing repetition will usually demonstrate inferior performance by aphasic patients. Naming tasks will clearly reveal aphasic patients' language problems by their production of paraphasic errors. The aphasic patient who is shown a key may say, "Pel, klo, klep, kleep . . . key," whereas the schizophrenic patient may call it a "key sort of watching tower thing." In this instance, the schizophrenic patient correctly identified the object, but incorporated it into his disordered thought process. Delirious or demented patients usually will have some naming trouble but not as severe as that seen in aphasic patients nor as bizarre as that seen in schizophrenic patients. When asked to name a key, the demented patient might well answer, "Lock, no . . . the lock keyer . . . key!"

The differential diagnosis of these conditions is important because a misdiagnosis may lead to gross mismanagement. For example, a very robust 80-year-old retired grocer began answering questions inappropriately at dinner one evening. Becoming concerned, his wife continued to ask questions, which the husband was unable to answer appropriately. He became frustrated, angry, and agitated. The wife became frightened and called the police. Because of this aggressive behavior, the man was jailed for 3 days. He was then transferred to a psychiatric hospital, where he remained for an additional 3 days before a neurologist diagnosed a Wernicke's aphasia secondary to a middle cerebral artery thrombosis. Mistakes such as this can be made unless a careful mental status examination is performed.

Differentiating the demented from the schizophrenic patient is usually not difficult because of the age difference, differences in behavior, and distinct differences in verbal output. On complete examination, additional data may corroborate the initial opinion. The demented patient may show problems with praxis and drawing. The schizophrenic patient often distorts drawings but usually can make recognizable copies of designs and figures. Ideational apraxia (see Chapter 9), which can be demonstrated by asking the patient to fold a letter and place it in an envelope, is often present in the demented patient but not in the schizophrenic patient.

Nonorganic Speech and Language Disorders

Several types of functional speech disorders can be mistaken for organic language patterns. Some neurotic patients will convert anxiety into a halting, effortful, telegraphic speech pattern (e.g., "Me want go home see wife"). These patients have normal comprehension, repetition, and naming but reduced verbal fluency. Reading and writing are also intact but are carried out in the same slow, effortful fashion. Mild dysarthria may also be present. These patients may require the help of both psychiatrists and speech pathologists to alter their speech patterns.

Other functional patients develop an acute aphonia (total inability to adduct the vocal cords and make audible sounds). Aphonia may arise as a pure conversion symptom or, more commonly, as a sequela to an insult to the speech apparatus. One middle-aged patient remained aphonic for 2 months after awakening from surgery with an endotracheal tube in place. Aphonic patients breathe normally and show no evidence of stridor (a sign of vocal cord paralysis). They communicate well by gesture, mouthing words, and writing. This type of functional overlay is well known to speech pathologists and responds well to therapy.

Elective mutism is another functional speech disorder that may be seen in both children and emotionally disturbed adults. It is characterized by a willful reluctance or an outright refusal to speak. The disorder may be complete (i.e., an absolute lack of speech in all situations) or relative (i.e., selective communication with a small circle of intimates). The speech, when present, may be limited to a mouthing of words; whispering; or a slow, labored, halting production. The electively mute adult typically has no language deficit and is physiologically capable of producing speech sounds. Some patients, especially children, do have a basic organic language disorder with considerable emotional overlay. The mutism is often resistant to the usual forms of speech therapy and psychotherapy[35] but can respond to behavior modification.[33]

SUMMARY

Language is a very complex and interesting higher-cognitive function. Because of the unique relationship of language and cerebral dominance, most acquired language disorders are pathognomonic of left hemisphere damage. Careful evaluation of language functions can localize the lesion within the dominant hemisphere. Language is of critical importance for many other cognitive functions; thus, the subsequent parts of the mental status examination must be administered and interpreted with some caution in aphasic patients.

REFERENCES

1. Albert ML: Language in normal and dementing elderly. In Obler, LV and Albert, ML (eds): Language and Communication in the Elderly. Lexington Books, Lexington, MA, 1980, pp 145–150.
2. Albert, ML, et al: Clinical Aspects of Dysphasia. Springer-Verlag, Vienna, 1981, pp 88–91.
3. Basso, A, Lecours, AR, Moraschini, S, et al: Anatomoclinical correlations of the aphasias as defined through computerized tomography: Exceptions. Brain Lang 26:201, 1985.
4. Benson, DF: Fluency in aphasia: Correlation with radioactive scan localization. Cortex 3:373, 1967.
5. Benson, DF: Psychiatric aspects of aphasia. Br J Psychiatr 123:555, 1973.
6. Benson, DF and Geschwind, N: Cerebral dominance and its disturbances. Pediatr Clin North Am 15:759, 1968.
7. Benson, DF and Zaias, BW: Progressive aphasia: A case with postmortem correlation. Neuropsychol Behav Neurol 4:215, 1991.
8. Bogan, J: Wernicke's area: Where is it? Thoughts about (and against) cortical localization. Paper presented at the 13th Annual Meeting of the Academy of Aphasia. Victoria, British Columbia, October 5, 1975.
9. Bogousslavsky, J, Regli, F, and Assal G: Acute transcortical mixed aphasia: A carotid occlusion syndrome with pial and watershed infarcts. Brain 111:631, 1988.
10. Borkowski, JG, Benton, AL, and Spreen, O: Word fluency and brain damage. Neuropsychologia 5:135, 1967.
11. Brown, JW and Hécaen, H: Lateralization and language representation. Neurology 26:183, 1976.
12. Caramazza, A: The logic of neuropsychological research and the problem of patient classification in aphasia. Brain Lang 21:9, 1984.
13. Cummings, JL and Benson, DF: Dementia: A Clinical Approach. Butterworth & Co, Boston, 1983.
14. Damasio, AR: Aphasia. N Engl J Med 326:531, 1992.
15. Damasio, AR, et al: Aphasia with nonhemorrhagic lesions in the basal ganglia and internal capsule. Arch Neurol 39:15, 1982.
16. Damasio, H and Damasio, AR: The anatomical basis of conduction aphasia. Brain 103:337, 1980.

17. Dejerine, J: Des differentes varietes de cecite verbale. Mémoires de la Société de Biologie 1892, pp 1–30.
18. Geschwind, N: Disconnection syndromes in animals and man. II. Brain 88:585, 1965.
19. Geschwind, N: Current concepts in aphasia. N Engl J Med 284:654, 1971.
20. Geschwind, N, Galaburda, AM: Cerebral Dominance: The biological foundations. Harvard University Press, Cambridge, MA, 1984.
21. Geschwind, N, Quadfasel, F, and Segarra, J: Isolation of the speech area. Neuropsychologia 6:327, 1968.
22. Gloning, I, et al: Comparison of verbal behavior in right-handed and non-right-handed patients with anatomically verified lesions of one hemisphere. Cortex 5:43, 1969.
23. Gloning, K: Handedness and aphasia. Neuropsychologia 15:355, 1977.
24. Goodglass, H and Kaplan, E: The Assessment of Aphasia and Related Disorders, ed 2. Lea & Febiger, Philadelphia, 1983.
25. Hécaen, H and de Ajuriaguerra, J: Left Handedness: Manual Superiority and Cerebral Dominance. Grune & Stratton, New York, 1964.
26. Luria, AR: On quasi-aphasia speech disturbances in lesions of the deep structures of the brain. Brain Lang 4:432, 1977.
27. Mendez, MF and Zander, BA: Dementia presenting with aphasia: Clinical characteristics. J Neurol Neurosurg Psychiatry 54:542, 1991.
28. Metter, EJ, et al: Comparison of metabolic rates, language and memory in subcortical aphasias. Brain Lang 19:33, 1983.
29. Metter, EJ, Kemple, D, Jackson, E, et al: Cerebral glucose metabolism in Wernicke's, Broca's and conduction aphasia. Arch Neurol 46:27, 1989.
30. Mohr, JP: Broca's area and Broca's aphasia. In Whitaker, H and Whitaker, H (eds): Studies in Neurolinguistics, Vol 1, Perspectives in Neurolinguistics and Psycholinguistics. Academic Press, New York, 1976, pp 201–235.
31. Mohr, JP, Watters, WC, and Duncan, AW: Thalamic hemorrhage and aphasia. Brain Lang 2:3, 1975.
32. Naeser, MA, et al: Aphasia with predominantly subcortical lesion sites: Description of three capsular/putaminal aphasia syndromes. Arch Neurol 39:2, 1982.
33. Norman, A and Broman, H: Volume feedback and generalization techniques in shaping speech of an electively mute boy: A case study. Percept Mot Skills 31:463, 1970.
34. Ojemann, G, et al: Cortical language localization in left dominant hemisphere: An electrical stimulation mapping investigation in 117 patients. J Neurosurg 71:316, 1989.
35. Reed, G: Elective mutism in children: A re-appraisal. J Child Psychol Psychiatry 4:99, 1963.
36. Rubens, AB and Kertesz, A: The localization of lesions in transcortical aphasias. In Kertesz, A (ed): Localization in Neuropsychology. Academic Press, New York, 1983, pp 245–268.
37. Strub, RL: Mental disorders in brain disease. In Frederiks, JAM (ed): Handbook of Clinical Neurology, Vol 2(46), Neurobehavioral Disorders. Elsevier, Amsterdam, 1985, pp 413–441.
38. Vargo, ME and Black, FW: Normative data for the Spreen-Benton Sentence Repetition Test. Cortex 20:585, 1984.
39. Vignolo, LA: Modality specific disorders of written language. In Kertesz, A (ed): Localization in Neuropsychology. Academic Press, New York, 1983, pp 357–369.
40. Wada, J: A new method for the determination of the side of cerebral speech dominance: A preliminary report on the intracarotid injection of sodium amytal in man. Med Biol 14:221, 1949.
41. Wilson, RS, Kaszniak, AW, and Fox, JH: Remote memory in senile dementia. Cortex 17:41, 1981.
42. Zangwill, OL: Two cases of crossed aphasia in dextrals. Neuropsychologia 17:167, 1979.

Chapter 6

Memory

Disturbances in memory are the most common complaint in patients with an organic mental syndrome. Almost all patients with dementia show memory problems early in the course of their disease. They may lose track of the date, forget work details, or fail to remember commitments that fall outside of their daily routines. In dementia the problem is insidious and can make it difficult or impossible for the patient to function effectively. There can be devastating effects on social and vocational adjustment before the organic nature of the problem is fully appreciated. Recognition of this memory difficulty allows the clinician and the family to help the patient avoid potential personal catastrophe. Careful attention to memory testing can often demonstrate the presence of an organic disorder before abnormal findings are noted on standard neurologic examination.

Various organic diseases result in different types of memory disturbance (e.g., severe memory deficit in relative isolation in Korsakoff's syndrome, memory difficulty compounded by inattention and agitation in the confusional states, or impaired recent memory associated with general cognitive dysfunction in dementia). In each of these diseases, memory is disturbed by different pathophysiological mechanisms.

Not all memory difficulties are organic in origin. Depressed and anxious patients, as well as other patients with significant psychiatric disorders, often have difficulty with memory. Because performance on memory testing requires maximum patient cooperation and effort, the emotionally disturbed patient will often perform poorly. The misdiagnosis of depression as dementia or the reverse is a serious diagnostic error that can lead to months or even years of inappropriate treatment. Untangling the memory problems in patients with a psychiatric disorder is difficult; however, full neurologic, psychiatric, and psychologic evaluation can almost always lead to the appropriate diagnosis. The diagnostic challenge is even greater when an organic problem such as early Alzheimer's disease is compounded by a superimposed depression or anxiety.

TERMINOLOGY

Memory is a general term for a mental process that allows the individual to store information for recall at a later time.[28] The time span for recall can be as short as a few seconds, as in a digit repetition task, or as long as many years, as in the recall of childhood experiences. The memory process consists of several stages. In the first, the information is received and registered by a particular sensory modality (e.g., touch, auditory, or visual). Once the sensory input has been received and registered, that information is held temporarily in short-term memory (working memory). The second step consists of storing or retaining the information in a more permanent form (long-term memory). This storage process is enhanced by repetition or by association with other information that is already in storage.[21] Storage is an active process that requires effort through practice and rehearsal.[19] The final step in the memory process is the recall or retrieval of the stored information. The retrieval step is an active process of mobilizing stored information. Each stage in the total memory process relies on the integrity of the previous steps. Any interruption in the hierarchy may prevent the storage or retrieval of a memory. Formal studies of memory have demonstrated that each aspect of memory involved separate yet interlocking neurobiologic substrates or systems; different diseases have differential effects on these systems and therefore produce various clinical pictures.

Clinically, memory is subdivided into three basic types based on the time span between stimulus presentation and memory retrieval. The terms *immediate, recent,* and *remote* are commonly used to denote these basic memory types. Unfortunately these terms are descriptive, and the time span implied is not well defined in clinical use. *Immediate memory* or immediate recall refers to the recall of a memory trace after an interval of a few seconds, as in repetition of a series of digits. The term *short-term memory* is also used by some to describe the task when the interval is filled with a distractor such as counting backward.

Recent memory refers to the patient's capacity to remember current, day-to-day events (e.g., the date, the doctor's name, what was eaten for breakfast, or recent news events). More strictly defined, recent memory is the ability to learn new material and to retrieve that material after an interval of minutes, hours, or days.

Remote memory is traditionally used to refer to the recollection of facts or events that occurred years previously, such as the names of teachers and old school friends, birth dates, and historic facts. In patients with a specific defect in new learning (recent memory), remote memory refers to the recall of events that occurred before the onset of the recent memory defect.

Amnesia generally describes a defect in memory function. Although applied to a broad spectrum of memory defects, amnesia is used most commonly to label patients with severe and relatively isolated memory deficits (e.g., Korsakoff's syndrome or posttraumatic amnesia). The inability to learn new material *after* the brain insult is called anterograde amnesia. Retrograde amnesia refers to amnesia for events that occurred *before* a brain insult. The period of amnesia may be as short as a few seconds or as long as several years. It is most commonly seen with head trauma but may also follow any major brain insult (e.g., stroke). Amnesia also refers to psychogenic amnesia, in which the patient blocks out a period of time. These patients do not demonstrate a recent memory deficit, can learn items during the amnestic period, and, after the amnestic period is over, do not have a defect in recent memory when tested. Psychologically based memory loss leaves patients with holes or relative holes in their memory for the events that occurred during the amnestic period. At times patients will recall parts of the amnestic period that were not emotionally traumatic yet will block the traumatic events.

EVALUATION

In the comprehensive mental status examination, each of the aspects of memory should be assessed in some detail. This will allow the examiner to distinguish the type of memory deficit (if any), the degree of memory loss, and the impact of the memory deficit on the patient's ability to function in a vocational or social role.

The patient will commonly show different performance levels on various memory tests, depending on the nature of the disorder (e.g., the patient with Korsakoff's syndrome will be able to respond very adequately to questions regarding more remote events but will be unable to learn new material). The use of several different memory tests is also of clinical importance. Brain-damaged patients will demonstrate differences in the incidence, nature, and degree of memory deficits based on the type of test used and the nature and location of their lesions.[2,3,8,14]

The accurate assessment of memory requires that any question asked by the examiner be verifiable from a source other than the patient. For example, it does very little good to ask patients when they graduated from high school or what they ate for lunch if the examiner cannot ascertain the accuracy of the patients' responses. Many patients with readily demonstrable memory deficits will deny their problem and may produce confabulated answers. Such responses may appear perfectly appropriate to the naive examiner who is unable to verify their accuracy. Personal information concerning the patient's social history, lifestyle, vocation, and so forth should be verified by the patient's family or friends.

Historic facts (e.g., "When was World War II?" or "Who was the president before Mr. Clinton?") are commonly used by examiners to screen both remote and recent memory. The basic knowledge of such information is closely related to the patient's basic premorbid intellectual level, education, and general social exposure. These factors must be assessed when considering the use of historic facts to test memory. If used at all, questions related to historic material must be tailored to the patient's background.

The most sensitive and valid tests of recent memory are those that require the patient to learn new material and recall it over time. The use of this technique eliminates some of the dangers of using unverified material and unknown social background. New learning is an active memory process that requires more expenditure of effort on the patient's part than does the mere recall of personal or historic facts.

When evaluating memory, the examiner must be aware of a number of more basic processes that can result in impaired performance even in the patient without an organic memory deficit. Performance on memory tests requires sustained attention. Accordingly, inattentive, distractible patients, regardless of etiology, will be unable to perform optimally on such tests. Patients in an acute confusional state or with a severe psychogenic disorder usually have impaired attention, which hinders memory performance. Disturbances of basic sensory, motor, or language functions that interfere with comprehension or expression will also result in impaired memory test performance. Poor memory performance by deaf, aphasic, acutely confused, psychotic, anxious, depressed, or grossly inattentive patients very well may reflect defects in these processes and should not be misinterpreted as evidence of specific, underlying stable memory deficits. Valid memory testing presumes that the patient is reasonable attentive, is capable of relating to and cooperating with the examiner, and has no defect that impairs the comprehension or expression of language.

Because of the clinical and social importance of memory, we have selected a number of memory tests that enable the examiner to assess a variety of memory processes. Many patients become apprehensive when having their memory tested, so it is important to present the material slowly and in as calm and nonthreatening a fashion as possible.

Immediate Recall (Short-Term Memory)

Immediate recall is usually tested by digit repetition. As this is covered in detail in Chapter 4, it will not be repeated here. Although backward digit repetition has been used by some examiners to assess verbal memory, this is a highly complex task that requires several neuropsychologic processes in addition to memory.[4] It is useful as a general screening test for brain dysfunction but should not be considered a test of short-term memory in isolation.

Orientation

The patient's orientation with respect to person (who he or she is), time (the date), and place (where he or she is) is important preliminary information and should be evaluated early in the examination of memory functioning.

Orientation to place and time are actually measures of recent memory, as they test the patient's ability to learn these continuing changes. If a patient is not fully oriented, this alone suggests a significant recent memory deficit.

Directions: The patient should be asked the following questions in sequence. Questions may be paraphrased when necessary to ensure clarity. If the patient fails these items, tell the patient the correct answers and have him or her repeat them; several minutes later, have the patient recall the answers. Failure at this level verifies very poor new learning ability and will predict deficient performance on any subsequent memory tasks.

1. Person
   a. Name   What is your name?
   b. Age   How old are you?
   c. Birth date   When is your birthday?
                          (day, month, year)

2. Place
   a. Location   Where are we right now?
                          What is the name of this place?
                          What kind of place are we in now?
                          What floor did you come to today?

   b. City location   What city are we in now?
                          State? County?

   c. Address   What is your home address?

3. Time
   a. Date   What is today's date?
                          (year, month, date)

   b. Day of the week   What day of the week is it?
   c. Time of day   What time is it right now?
   d. Season of the year What season is it now?

Normal people perform perfectly on this test, although somewhat less adequate scores are noted on time orientation by some individuals.[24] The only orientation items that are sometimes failed by normal individuals are the exact date of the month and, less commonly, the day of the week. Performance correlates with education level; college graduates, if they do not know the exact date or day, usually miss by only one day, whereas normal people without a high school education may miss by 2 or even 3 days.[18] A small number (7.7%) of uneducated individuals may incorrectly identify the month.

Remote Memory

Tests in this section evaluate the patient's ability to recall events of both a personal and historic nature. As emphasized, personal events must be verifiable by a reliable source other than the patient; the performance on the recall of historic information must be interpreted in light of the patient's premorbid intelligence, education, and social experience.

1. Personal information
   a. Where were you born?
   b. School information: Where did you go to school?

      When did you attend school?

      Where is your school located?
   c. Vocation history: What do you do for work?

      Where have you worked?

      When did you work at those places?
   d. Family information: What is your wife's (children's) name?

      How old is your wife (children)?

      What was your mother's maiden name?

Personal information items are completed with approximately equal accuracy by both normal patients and patients with mild, nonspecific brain damage. Although impaired performance is pathologic, this test does not efficiently differentiate between groups.[24]

2. Historic facts
   a. Ask the patient to name four people who have been president during the patient's lifetime. The normal patient should be able to accomplish this task without difficulty. A slightly more difficult task, and one that is very frequently failed by patients with early Alzheimer's disease, is asking the patient to name the last four or five presidents in proper reverse sequence, starting with the current president.
   b. Ask the patient to name the last war in which the United States was directly involved. At the time of this writing, the correct response would be the war in Iraq (Desert Storm). An older patient may name the Vietnam War, Korean War, or World War II. If the patient gives one of these responses, ask him or her about any recollection of the Iraq war. If the patient has no memory for these major events, this implies deficient memory.

New-Learning Ability

This section assesses the patient's ability to actively learn new material (to acquire new memories). Adequate performance requires the integrity of the total memory system: recognition and registration of the initial sensory input, retention and storage of the information, and recall or retrieval of the stored information. An interruption in any of these stages will impair clinically relevant new-learning ability. A careful clinical examination of how the patient fails a particular task may often provide valuable information as to the nature of the impaired process. Patients with impaired memory, particularly patients with Alzheimer's disease, can become rather overwhelmed during this extensive memory testing. Items previously presented inhibit and confuse learning on subsequent items (proactive interference). In such situations, the patients may provide answers from earlier test items in later testing. These intrusion errors are characteristic of many organic syndromes, especially dementia.

Four Unrelated Words

Directions: Tell the patient, "I am going to tell you four words that I would like you to remember. In a few minutes, I will ask you to recall these words." To ensure that the patient has heard, understood, and initially retained the four words, have him or her repeat the words after their presentation. Correct any errors made on immediate repetition. Older patients (greater than age 75) may require several trials to learn the words, but when a patient must be given four or five trials to repeat the words accurately, this usually forecasts a significant memory problem. To eliminate possible mental rehearsal, interference should be used between presentation and recall of the words. Accordingly, the examiner may wish to present the four words before the remote memory or orientation examination. After 5 minutes, ask for the recall of the four words. Information concerning the duration of memory can be obtained by asking for a recall of the word after 10 and 30 minutes. The following words have been selected because of their semantic and phonemic diversity.

TEST ITEMS

1. Brown	1. Fun
2. Honesty	2. Carrot
3. Tulip	3. Ankle
4. Eyedropper	4. Loyalty

When a patient is unable to recall a word, it is often possible to obtain an indication of memory storage by the use of verbal cues. These include semantic cues relating to the category of the named object (e.g., "one word was a color"), phonemic cues using syllabic components of the word (e.g., "Hon . . . [honesty]"), and contextual cues (e.g., "A common flower in Holland is _____"). If a patient is unable to either spontaneously recall the words or to recall them with cues, the examiner may resort to asking the patient if he or she recognizes the appropriate word from a series of words (e.g., "Was the color red, green, brown, or yellow?"). Significantly better recognition than spontaneous recall suggests that the memory problem is due to a retrieval defect rather than an acquisition or storage deficit.

Scoring: The normal patient under age 60 is expected to accurately recall three or four of the words after a 10-minute delay.[24] There is a significant variation within the normal population on this test (standard deviation 0.8 words), however, so the clinical implication of a low score (e.g., 2 of 4) must be interpreted in light of the patient's history and the performance on the entire examination. As demonstrated in Table 6–1, there is an age-related decline in performance on this test in normal individuals over 60 years of age. Octogenarians average only two of four words retained over 5 minutes, with a substantial variance. They will improve their performance at 10 and 30 minutes after being reminded of the correct words. Patients with dementia, on the other hand, do not improve on subsequent trials (see Table 6–1).

Table 6–1. RECENT MEMORY PERFORMANCE*

	NORMAL INDIVIDUALS (AGE IN YEARS)					ALZHEIMER'S DISEASE PATIENTS (STAGE)			
	40–49	50–59	60–69	70–79	80–89	I	II	III	IV
4 Words									
5 min	3.1	2.9	2.0	1.8	2.1	1.6	0.4	0	0
	(0.9)	(1.3)	(1.0)	(0.8)	(1.4)	(1.2)	(0.7)	(0.1)	
10 min	3.7	3.5	3.0	2.6	2.7	1.9	0.7	0.1	0
	(0.7)	(0.8)	(1.0)	(0.9)	(1.4)	(1.4)	(1.0)	(0.4)	
30 min	3.7	4.0	3.5	3.1	2.9	1.8	0.6	0.1	0
	(0.7)	(0.0)	(0.7)	(1.2)	(1.1)	(1.4)	(1.0)	(0.3)	
Story	10.1	11.1	9.7	8.2	7.6	5.5	2.8	0.6	0
	(2.8)	(1.9)	(2.6)	(3.3)	(2.8)	(2.3)	(2.0)	(1.0)	
5 Objects	4.6	4.7	4.2	3.9	3.8	2.3	1.1	0.2	0
	(0.6)	(0.6)	(0.8)	(1.0)	(1.6)	(1.7)	(1.3)	(0.5)	
Paired Associate Learning (Both Trials)									
Easy	3.8	3.8	3.6	3.1	3.6	3.2	2.4	0.8	0
	(0.4)	(0.6)	(0.7)	(1.2)	(0.7)	(0.7)	(0.9)	(1.1)	
Difficult	3.3	3.2	2.6	2.1	2.3	1.7	0.9	0.1	0
	(1.0)	(0.7)	(1.3)	(1.0)	(1.0)	(0.9)	(1.0)	(0.4)	

*Mean and standard deviation, n = 100.

Verbal Story for Immediate Recall

Directions: Tell the patient, "I am going to read you a short paragraph. Listen carefully, because when I finish reading, I want you to tell me everything that I told you." In older patients, read the story more slowly to give them adequate time to process the information. After reading the story, say "Now tell me everything that you can remember of the story. Start at the beginning of the story and tell me all that happened." The separate items in the story are indicated by slash (/) marks. As the patient retells the story, indicate the number of ideas recalled. In patients with good immediate recall, it may be useful to ask for another recall after 30 minutes. This is a sensitive method of assessing short-term verbal recall.

Test Item

It was July / and the Rogers / had packed up / their four children / in the station wagon / and were off / on vacation.

They were taking / their yearly trip / to the beach / at Gulf Shores. / This year / they were making / a special 1-day stop / at the Aquarium / in New Orleans.

After a long day's drive / they arrived / at the motel / only to discover / that in their excitement / they had left / the twins / and their suitcases / in the front yard.

Scoring: The story contains 26 relatively separate ideas or information bits. In our experience, the normal individual under age 70 should be expected to produce at least 10 of these items on immediate recall. In the 70s, the average score drops to 8.2, and in the 80s, to 7.6. Elderly individuals are slower in their auditory processing and are less able to store as much information on a single presentation as are younger people. Less adequate performance than this by the nonretarded patient indicates defective verbal recall ability. Story recall significantly discriminates between brain-damaged and low-IQ normal groups and also between normal individuals and Alzheimer patients (see Tables 6–1 and 6–2).

Visual Memory (Hidden Objects)

Directions: Visual memory testing should be used with all patients, but it is especially useful in evaluating the memory of aphasic patients. This test item is also very good for patients with reduced verbal abilities or lack of education. The examiner may use any five small, easily recognizable objects that may be readily hidden in the patient's vicinity. We commonly use items such as a pen, comb, keys, coin, and fork. The use of five items provides a reasonable span for most patients. The objects are hidden while the patient is watching. Name each item as it is hidden to

Table 6–2. STATISTICAL COMPARISON OF MEMORY TESTS

Variable	Brain Damaged Mean	Low-IQ Normal Mean	F
Total score	33.4	50.0	28.0‡
Digit repetition	4.2	4.8	1.9
Vigilance errors	10.2	0.2	5.5†
Orientation	8.7	10.6	13.3‡
Person	2.6	3.0	7.5‡
Place	2.7	3.0	3.4*
Time	3.4	4.6	8.4‡
Remote memory			
Personal information	3.4	3.9	3.1
Historic facts	1.3	1.5	3.2
Four words—10 min	1.9	3.6	15.1‡
Four words—30 min	1.8	3.9	20.4‡
Visual memory			
Hidden objects found (4)	1.3	3.7	10.8‡
Hidden objects named	1.0	0.2	3.1
Paired associate learning			
Easy	2.1	3.0	12.6‡
Difficult	1.4	3.0	9.7‡
Total	3.5	6.0	15.6‡

* $P < .05$.
† $P < .01$.
‡ $P < .001$.

ensure that the patient is aware of which object was hidden in what place. After hiding the objects, the examiner should provide interfering stimuli by administering another mental status task, asking the patient routine questions, or engaging the patient in general conversation. An interference period of 5 minutes should suffice. After this period, ask the patient to name and indicate the location of each of the hidden objects. If the patient is unable to recall the location of any object, ask him or her to name the hidden object.

Scoring: The average patient under 60 should find four or five (4.6 ± 0.6) of the hidden objects after a 5-minute delay without difficulty. Older patients (age 70 to 90) will not do quite as well (3.8 ± 1.3). Less adequate performance (fewer than three objects) indicates impaired usual memory. A patient with aphasia should be able to find the objects but may not be able to name them.

Visual Memory (Visual Design Reproduction)

This is a part of most memory batteries, and it is a very useful test item but can be considered optional and is not usually used as a component of a routine mental status examination. It is not a test of visual memory alone because problems with constructional ability (see Chapter 7) will also adversely affect performance. Several examples of such tests are listed in Appendix 1.

Directions: The following subtest uses four simple line drawings of increasing complexity. We recommend that the examiner provide standardized stimuli cards to ensure uniformity, although the examiner may choose to draw each design at the bedside. The patient is required to reproduce each of the four designs on a piece of white paper after a 5-second presentation of the design and a 10-second delay before beginning. The following instructions are given: "I am now going to show you some simple drawings. I want you to look at each drawing as I show it to you. Be sure to look at it carefully so that you can draw what you have seen from memory. Do not draw the design until I have told you to begin." (Fig. 6–1).

Scoring: Each design may be scored on a four-point scale, with values from 0 to 3. The higher the score, the more adequate the reproduction. The following scoring system may be used to aid the examiner in quantifying performance on this test:

0—Poor	Given for a failure to recall and reproduce the design
1—Fair	Given for recognizable but distorted, rotated, partially omitted, or confabulated features of the design
2—Good	Given for easily recognizable designs with minor errors of integration, omission, or addition
3—Excellent	Given for perfect (or near perfect) reproductions of the items with all appropriate components, placements, and integration

Representative clinical examples of poor, fair, good, and excellent drawings are shown in Figures 6–2 through 6–5, to aid the examiner in rating each design.

The average patient should produce reproductions of each design at the 2 and 3 scoring levels. All designs should be recalled. Less adequate performance indicates a deficit in visual memory.

Paired Associate Learning

Paired associate learning (PAL) is commonly used in standard memory batteries and is another highly sensitive measure of new-learning ability.

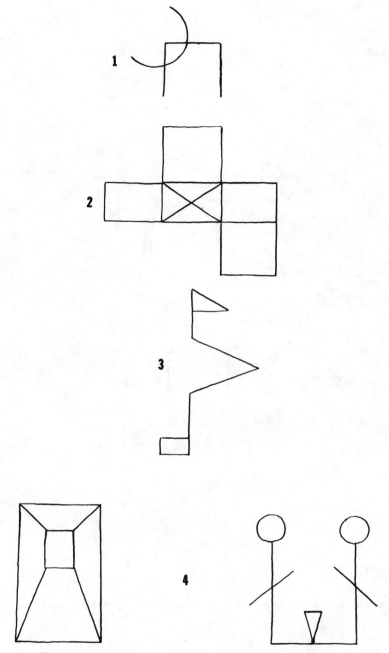

Figure 6–1. Test items for Visual Design Reproduction Test.

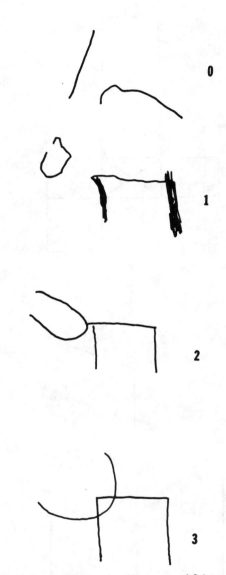

Figure 6–2. Renderings of design 1, with scores of 0 (poor) through 3 (excellent).

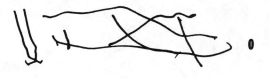

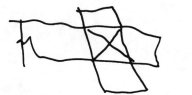

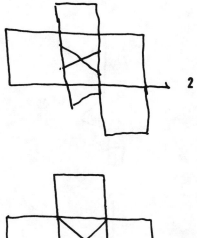

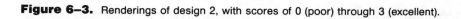

Figure 6–3. Renderings of design 2, with scores of 0 (poor) through 3 (excellent).

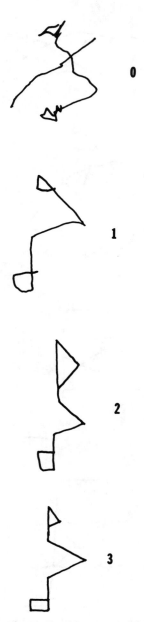

Figure 6–4. Renderings of design 3, with scores of 0 (poor) through 3 (excellent).

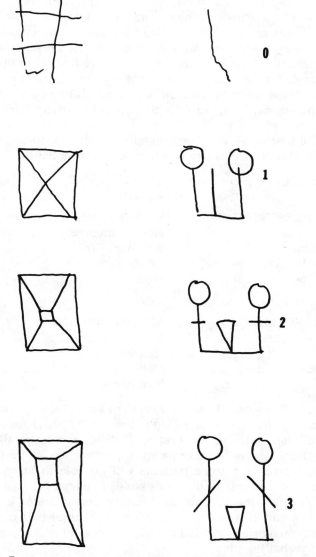

Figure 6–5. Renderings of design 4, with scores of 0 (poor) through 3 (excellent).

Directions: Tell the patient, "I am going to read you a list of words, two at a time. Listen carefully because I will expect you to remember the words that go together. For example, if the words were big—little, I would expect you to say the word 'little' after I said the word 'big.' " When the patient is clear as to the directions, continue as follows: "Now listen carefully to the words as I read them." Read the first presentation at the rate of one pair every 2 seconds. After reading the first presentation, test for recall by presenting the first recall list. Give the first word of a pair and allow 5 seconds for a response. If the patient gives a correct response, say "That's right" and proceed with the next pair. If the patient gives an incorrect response, say "No," provide the correct word, and proceed to the next pair.

After the first recall has been completed, allow a 10-second interval and give the second presentation list, proceeding as before.

TEST ITEMS
PRESENTATION LISTS

FIRST PRESENTATION	**SECOND PRESENTATION**
Weather—Box	House—Income
High—Low	Weather—Box
House—Income	Book—Page
Book—Page	High—Low

RECALL LISTS

FIRST RECALL	**SECOND RECALL**
House—_____	Book—_____
High—_____	House—_____
Weather—_____	High—_____
Book—_____	Weather—_____

Scoring: The normal patient less than age 70 is expected to recall the two "easy" paired associates (high—low, book—page) and at least one of the "hard" associates of the first recall trial, and to recall all paired associates on the second trial. In patients greater than 70, performance is slightly less adequate.[22] Some patients will be able to learn the paired words with strong natural associations but will be unable to learn the pairs without such associations. This discrepancy demonstrates a reliance on semantic cues and an inability to learn new material that cannot be associated with memories already in storage. The total PAL score is the best measure of verbal learning.

The results of a statistical comparison of these memory tests between 25 patients with mixed brain damage and 25 normal patients with IQs less than 80 appear in Table 6–2. Differences in age and education were controlled.[24]

CLINICAL IMPLICATIONS

Some aspects of the memory process are associated with certain neuroanatomic structures or neuronal systems. Pathologic studies have amply documented that limbic structures are involved in the long-term storage and retrieval of recent information.[6,17,22,31] However, the structures that are required for immediate recall and remote memory are not as well established. Although all memory traces—visual, verbal, and tactile—are most likely stored in the neocortex, many subcortical structures are necessary for the total memory process (registration, storage, and retrieval). Damage or disruption of different cortical or subcortical systems will result in varied patterns of dysfunction.

Immediate Recall

The immediate recall of digits is a process that does not require any long-term storage of information, but it does require initial registration, short-term holding, and verbal repetition. This entire process can be performed by the language cortex surrounding the sylvian fissure. This has been demonstrated in patients with transcortical aphasia.[11] The exact mechanism by which these short-term memories are maintained within the language system is not known. Reverberating circuits may be established, or patterns of cortical after-image may be present. Whatever change does occur, it is not long-lasting. Efficient short-term memory is not a passive process, and there are several factors that favor good performance. A digit sequence task will be performed much better if active mental rehearsal can take place. Also, if the patient actively groups digits into two- or three-digit sets, performance will be improved. A third and always very important element in all memory processing is the association of the new material with previously stored information; for example, a digit sequence that is similar to an old phone number or address will be much more easily recalled than a completely unique random sequence. Short-term memory (immediate recall) is a distinct property of the cortical sensory, motor, and integrative areas necessary to register, recall, and produce the original stimulus. It does not require the limbic systems necessary for long-term storage and permanent memory formation.

If there is any damage to or disruption of these basic sensory or motor areas, then short-term memory will be faulty. In digit repetition, the language system is essential; therefore, any degree of aphasia (excluding the transcortical aphasias) can cause disruption of immediate memory functioning. This repetition failure is particularly pronounced in conduction aphasia.[30] The primary deficit in conduction aphasia is an inability to repeat. Whether this repetition failure is a defect in language or short-term memory is an open question that may, in fact, reflect an argument of semantics.

Probably the most common cause of failure on short-term memory tasks is inattention.[25] If a patient's attention strays from the stimulus during presentation, the information may be imperfectly registered. Similarly, if the patient is inattentive during the repetition phase and time pauses occur, the memory trace will fade. Inattention can be organic, as in confusional states and dementia, or functional, as in anxiety and depression.

The demented patient will have difficulty with immediate memory for several reasons: such patients are often inattentive; they have cortical atrophy, which affects their basic language and other sensory-motor integration systems; and they have general intellectual deterioration.[33]

Recent Memory

In general, the ability to store and then retrieve new material (recent memory, new learning, or memorizing) presumes intact registration, retention, and short-term storage. If the material is familiar and can be associated with information already in long-term storage, the process is easier and relies less on short-term storage.[21]

Certain limbic structures are required to ensure storage and retrieval. The hippocampi, the mamillary bodies, and the dorsal medial nuclei of the thalami are essential subcortical links in the storage and retrieval of both verbal and nonverbal memories.[6,22,31] Actual memories are probably not stored in these structures, but the limbic system seems to act as the mechanism to store and retrieve memories from the cortex.

Whenever these subcortical structures are destroyed or severely damaged, the patient is rendered unable to learn new material (anterograde amnesia) or to retrieve memories from the recent past (retrograde amnesia). These patients literally become fixed in time and are unable to record the passing of events from that time onward. In certain clinical situations, these limbic structures are damaged in isolation. Such patients develop a profound organic amnesic state. This condition is characterized clinically by the following findings: (1) severe anterograde amnesia; (2) moderate to severe retrograde amnesia, which can extend back for several years; and, usually, (3) confabulation during the acute stage. In the face of this devastating memory impairment, such patients have remarkably intact immediate memory, as assessed by the Digit Repetition and other similar tests. These patients also demonstrate no change in premorbid levels of intelligence. They carry on coherent, intelligent conversations that appear abnormal only when recent events are discussed. Because these patients do not remember the date, place, and recent events, they may appear confused.

This dramatic organic amnesic state has been seen secondary to bilateral temporal lobectomy, herpes simplex encephalitis, and bilateral hippocampal infarction. In these cases, the hippocampus has been completely destroyed bilaterally. A similar memory deficit is seen clinically in Korsakoff's syndrome (a syndrome of thiamine depletion seen in chronic alcoholism and severe malnutrition). In Korsakoff's syndrome, the lesions involve bilateral destruction of the mamillary bodies and the dorsal medial nuclei of the thalami. The patient with Korsakoff's syndrome frequently, but not invariably, goes through an acute encephalopathy (Wernicke's encephalopathy) at the onset of the memory difficulty. Vascular or traumatic lesions of the dorsal medial thalamus also cause severe organic amnesia.[26,29]

In Alzheimer's dementia, patients also have defects in new learning. These defects are due in part to a gradual degeneration of the cells in the hippocampus as well as in the basal nucleus of Meynert. The memory loss in the atrophic dementias is more complex than that seen in the organic amnesias, and will be discussed more fully in the section that deals with remote memory.

The amnesia most familiar to the lay person is the memory loss that occurs after head injury. Patients with moderate to severe closed head injury almost always have some degree of retrograde amnesia for the time immediately preceding the injury, and they usually have transient difficulty learning new material after the trauma. In head trauma, the temporal lobes are commonly concussed against the bony confines of the middle fossa. This trauma causes a physiologic disruption of hippocampal function, which in turn disturbs memory storage and retrieval. Posttraumatic amnesia is usually reversible, but in cases of significant temporal lobe damage, the memory loss can be permanent. Repeated concussion, such as that seen in boxers, may result in gradual but permanent memory disturbance. An interesting feature of the amnesia seen with acute head injury is that the retrograde amnesic period will shorten in the days following recovery of consciousness. Initially the patient may not recall events that occurred years preceding the accident. Within several days, the patient may remember all but the few minutes that immediately preceded the accident. This shrinking retrograde amnesia verifies that the injury did not eliminate the memories from storage but merely rendered them temporarily irretrievable.[1,15]

Clinically, the memory disturbance in the various types of organic amnesias is similar (i.e., the patients cannot recall recent information). On experimental tasks, however, it has been shown that patients with Korsakoff's syndrome, whose damage is in the thalamus and mamillary body, have actually retained a considerable amount of the material presented to them, but are unaware of this (the memory is implicit but not explicit). The deficit is with retrieving the information and realizing that it has been presented, rather than with the storage process. Patients with hippocampal and temporal lobe damage have both a storage and a retrieval defect. As mentioned earlier, the fact that the cortex of the Korsakoff patient has stored the engrams for the memory does not help the patient clinically because he or she does not realize that they are stored and thus cannot retrieve and use the information.[32]

Transient global amnesia is another type of organic memory problem.[13] This syndrome probably involves transient ischemia of both medial temporal lobes secondary to decreased perfusion in the territory of the posterior cerebral arteries.[12,16] Single photon emission computerized tomography (SPECT) perfusion scans usually demonstrate this bilateral or unilateral left temporal lobe hypoperfusion. This syndrome is characterized by an acute, but temporary, confusional state with amnesia. The patients are disoriented to time and place and have a significant defect in new-learning ability. Fortunately, recovery generally occurs within hours or days, and the patient is left with a permanent amnesia only for the duration of the episode itself. Some patients, however, may experience permanent memory loss and demonstrate bilateral hippocampal infarction.[7] The following case illustrates some of the essential features of this syndrome:

> Dr. JL was a robust 68-year-old educator who was addressing a teacher's convention. In the middle of his speech, he stopped suddenly, became dazed, and began to ask where he was. He repeatedly asked, "What am I doing?" and "Where am I?" On initial neurologic examination, he was distraught and very confused. He was unable to attend well and was unable to learn new material. He did not remember arriving in New Orleans, but he did know that he was scheduled to attend the convention. One day later, his mental function was essentially normal except that he was amnesic for the day prior to and the day of his amnesic episode.

All of the conditions discussed thus far have resulted from bilateral lesions localized in limbic structures. Although it is true that a bilateral lesion is necessary to produce a profound memory loss, there is some loss of specific memory functions after a unilateral lesion. Unilateral dominant temporal lobectomy patients show a relative decrease in verbal learning, whereas patients with unilateral nondominant temporal lobectomies demonstrate a decrease in visual memory.[17] This pattern of differential deficits is also seen with unilateral subcortical lesions.[27]

Various factors other than specific limbic damage can interfere with the storage and retrieval of new material; some of these have been discussed in the previous section, but they merit additional mention here. Inattention will prevent any patient from accurately storing new material. Because efficient memory storage requires close attention to the information for short-term registration and storage, the results of memory testing in inattentive patients must be interpreted with caution. Aphasic patients are also at a tremendous disadvantage in any verbal learning task;

if they cannot accurately comprehend or repeat verbal material, it is not valid to judge their memory capacity using that material. Nonverbal memory tasks are necessary to assess validly memory in aphasic patients. Memory test performance and intelligence are directly related; accordingly, patients' premorbid intellectual levels must be considered when interpreting the results of memory testing. Deficits in basic sensory capacity (i.e., hearing and vision) are sometimes overlooked in testing, but obviously sensory systems must be adequate for memory testing in each specific modality.

The patient's emotional state can also significantly affect new-learning ability. Very anxious patients will make errors owing to inattention and distractibility. Depressed patients perform poorly on memory testing because of their inability to put forth the required effort to memorize the presented material.

Depressed patients also tend to remember negative or sad information more effectively than positive or happy events or ideas.[5] In significant depression, the decrease in motivation and learning probably involves more than purely psychologic mechanisms. The underlying chemical disorder postulated in major depressive disorders undoubtedly adversely affects neuronal functioning at various levels.[9]

Poor performance on memory tests is probably the single most important factor that may result in the misdiagnosis of depression as dementia.[20] Accordingly, in the patient with psychomotor retardation and memory problems, the diagnosis of depression must be considered and carefully pursued during the evaluation process.

Remote Memory

When a memory has remained in a persons' repertoire for a number of years, it can be considered a remote, or old, memory. These memories are stored in the appropriate association cortex (e.g., language cortex for verbal material). In contrast to recent memory, remote memory does not require the limbic system for retrieval from storage. Patients with Korsakoff's syndrome or bilateral temporal lobectomy can accurately discuss personal and historic events that occurred years previously (remote memory), yet they are unable to remember what they had for breakfast that morning (recent memory).[23] There is apparently a mechanism, thus far unexplained, by which memories finally become sufficiently well established that they can be recalled without the aid of subcortical limbic structures. These remote memories can be lost only by damage to the cortical storage areas themselves. This loss of remote, or old, memories is seen in patients with the atrophic dementias (Alzheimer's and Pick's) or those with any disease that damages extensive areas of the cortex. The memory disturbance in the demented patient is complex: such patients have difficulty with short-term memory because of atrophy in the basic sensory association cortex (e.g., language cortex for verbal memory); they are hampered in recent memory acquisition because of degeneration of cells in the basilar nucleus of Meynert and hippocampal system; and they have defects in remote memory because of widespread cortical atrophy.

Functional Memory Disturbances

Not all memory disorders are of organic origin, and knowledge of the functional disturbances of memory is important. The interference with memory performance that can occur secondary to anxiety and depression has been discussed previously. There are, however, several psychiatric conditions in which memory disturbances are central features. The first and most common is the dissociative state, now called psychogenic amnesia. This is the classic amnesia that has been popularized in the press and in movies. Such patients either lose their identity completely and travel to a new location (fugue or psychogenic fugue state), or have periods of minutes, hours, or days when they carry out their normal life routine and later become aware that they remember nothing of what transpired during this period (dissociative state). During a dissociative or fugue state, the patients do not usually act confused, as do persons with transient global amnesia, and they are able to learn new material, unlike patients with organic amnesia. There should be no difficulty in differentiating the organic amnesic, who cannot learn new material when tested, from the psychogenic amnesic who has experienced a "memory lapse." Brief testing using the four unrelated words task or the paired associate words task should suffice.

There is one other curious pseudomemory disturbance: Ganser's syndrome, or the syndrome of approximate answers. These patients will routinely give approximate answers to all questions: for example, today is Tuesday (actually it is Wednesday), the month is March (actually it is April), or 2 and 2 are 5. Because their answers are so consistently close to the correct answer, it is obvious that they have more knowledge of the subject in question than they are indicating. Although the approximate answer is the most characteristic symptom, Ganser's original patients all had clouded consciousness, hallucinations, and somatic conversion symptoms.[10]

The syndrome was originally described in prisoners, but it is not exclusively seen in this population. The syndrome is uncommon and is not typically seen in children. Its etiology is unclear, but some patients have a schizophrenic disorder or an underlying organic mental disorder. The nature and inconsistency of their mental status findings strongly suggest a significant component of either hysteria or malingering. Most patients have some motivating reason to appear legally insane, incompetent, or cognitively impaired.

On occasion, professed memory loss is a conscious and motivated symptom of malingering. It may be associated with other feigned neurologic or psychiatric symptoms but can also be seen alone. The patients whom we have seen usually have a very specific, well-recognized reason for their malingering (in our experience, either avoiding prosecution by virtue of incompetence, or gaining compensation for a minor head injury). On examination, these patients may give approximate answers or very bizarre answers. Their memory loss is usually inconsistent, in that they may fail all memory testing but remember a football score from the previous weekend. They also claim patches of remote memory loss and at times claim not to remember their own name.

SUMMARY

In general, memory is a hierarchic process in which information must first be registered in a basic sensory cortical area and then processed through the limbic system for new learning to occur. Finally, the material is permanently established in the appropriate association cortex. At this point, limbic retrieval is no longer required in the recall process. The immediate recall system is disturbed by damage to the primary sensory or motor cortex or by inattention. Learning is prevented by damage to the hippocampi or the dorsal medial thalamic nuclei. Old remote memories are resistant to limbic damage but will be lost when widespread cortical damage occurs. Careful testing of the various aspects of memory can frequently lead to both a clinical and an anatomic diagnosis.

REFERENCES

1. Benson, DF and Geschwind, N: Shrinking retrograde amnesia. J Neurol Neurosurg Psychiatry 30:539, 1967.
2. Benton, A and Spreen, O: Visual memory test performance in mentally deficient and brain-damaged patients. Am J Ment Defic 68:630, 1964.
3. Bisiach, E and Faglioni, P: Recognition of random shapes by patients with unilateral lesions as a function of complexity, association value, and delay. Cortex 10:101, 1974.
4. Black, FW and Strub, RL: Digit repetition performance in patients with focal brain damage. Cortex 14:12, 1978.
5. Breslow, R, Kocsis, J, and Belkin, B: Contribution of the depressive perspective to memory function in depression. Am J Psychiatry 138:227, 1981.
6. DeJong, R, Itabashi, HI, and Olson, J: Memory loss due to hippocampal lesions. Arch Neurol 20:339, 1969.
7. DeJong, R: The hippocampus and its role in memory. J Neurol Sci 19:73, 1973.
8. DeRenzi, E: Nonverbal memory and hemispheric side of lesion. Neuropsychologia 6:181, 1968.
9. Folstein, MF and McHugh, PP: Dementia syndrome of depression. In Katzman, R, Terry, RD, and Beck, KL (eds): Alzheimer's Disease: Senile Dementia and Related Disorders, Vol 7, Aging. Raven Press, New York, 1978, pp 87–94.
10. Ganser, SJM: A peculiar hysterical state. In Hirsch, SR and Shepherd, M (eds): Themes and Variations in European Psychiatry: An Anthology. J Wright, Bristol, 1974, pp 67–77.

11. Geschwind, N, Quadfasel, F, and Segarra, J: Isolation of the speech area. Neuropsychologia 67:327, 1968.
12. Heathfield, K, Croft, P, and Swash, M: The syndrome of transient global amnesia. Brain 96:729, 1973.
13. Hodges, JR and Warlow, CP: Syndromes of transient amnesia. J Neurol Neurosurg Psychiatry 53:834, 1990.
14. Lewinsohn, P, et al: A comparison between frontal and nonfrontal right and left hemisphere brain-damaged patients. J Comp Physiol Psychol 81:248, 1972.
15. Logan, W and Sherman, DG: Transient global amnesia. Stroke 14:1005, 1983.
16. Mathew, N and Meyer, J: Pathogenesis and natural history of transient global amnesia. Stroke 5:303, 1974.
17. Milner, B: Intellectual functions of the temporal lobes. Psychol Bull 51:42, 1954.
18. Natelson, BH, et al: Temporal orientation and education: A direct relationship in normal people. Arch Neurol 36:444, 1979.
19. Neisser, U: Cognitive Psychology. Appleton-Century-Crofts, New York, 1967.
20. Nott, P and Fleminger, J: Presenile dementia: The difficulties of early diagnosis. Acta Psychiatr Scand 51:210, 1975.
21. Parkin, AJ: Residual learning capability in organic amnesia. Cortex 18:417, 1982.
22. Scoville, W and Milner, B: Loss of recent memory after bilateral hippocampal lesions. J Neurol Neurosurg Psychiatry 20:11, 1957.
23. Selzer, B and Benson, DF: The temporal pattern of retrograde amnesia in Korsakoff's disease. Neurology 24:527, 1974.
24. Simpson, N, Black, FW, and Strub, RL: Memory assessment using the Strub-Black mental status exam and the Wechsler memory scale. J Clin Psychol 42:147, 1986.
25. Smith, A: The Serial Sevens Subtraction Test. Arch Neurol 17:78, 1967.
26. Speedie, LJ and Heilman, KM: Amnestic disturbances following infarction of the left dorsomedial nucleus of the thalamus. Neuropsychologia 20:597, 1982.
27. Speedie, LJ and Heilman, KM: Anterograde memory deficits for visuospatial material after infarction of the right thalamus. Neuropsychologia 40:183, 1983.
28. Squire, LR and Butters, N (eds): Neuropsychology of Memory. The Guilford Press, New York, 1984.
29. Squire, LR and Moore, RY: Dorsal thalamic lesion in a noted case of human memory dysfunction. Ann Neurol 6:503, 1979.
30. Strub, R and Gardner, H: The repetition defect in conduction aphasia: Mnestic or linguistic? Brain Lang 1:241, 1975.
31. Victor, M, Adams, R, and Collins, G: The Wernicke-Korsakoff Syndrome and Related Neurologic Disorders Due to Alcoholism and Malnutrition, ed 2. FA Davis, Philadelphia, 1989.
32. Warrington, EK and Weiskrantz, L: Amnesia: A disconnection syndrome. Neuropsychologia 20:233, 1982.
33. Wilson, R, et al: Primary memory and secondary memory in dementia of the Alzheimer type. J Clin Neuropsyhchol 5:337, 1983.

Chapter 7

Constructional Ability

Constructional tasks such as line drawings and block designs are extremely useful for detecting organic brain disease and should be included in every mental status examination. Constructional ability (constructional praxis) can be defined as the capacity to draw or construct two- or three-dimensional figures or shapes. Copying line drawings using pencil on paper, reproducing matchstick patterns, and reconstructing block designs are all examples of routinely used tests of constructional ability. This high-level, nonverbal cognitive function is a very complex perceptual motor task that involves an integration of occipital, parietal, and frontal lobe functions. Because of the extensive cortical area necessary to perform constructional tasks, early or subtle brain damage frequently disrupts performance. In some patients, the unsuccessful attempt to copy a simple line drawing can be the only objective evidence suggesting organic brain disease.

Despite their importance and proven clinical use, constructional tasks are frequently not included in bedside or office mental status testing, partly because very few patients actually complain of constructional impairment. Architects or engineers, whose professions require such abilities, might notice difficulty when drawing plans, reading blueprints, or translating plans into actual construction, but most patients are quite surprised to find that they are unable to draw a clock or copy a block design when asked to do so. Because constructional tests take only a few minutes to perform and can yield very valuable data, we encourage every clinician to use them.

The term "constructional ability," rather than the more classic term "constructional praxis," will be used to discuss this general area of cognitive function. Praxis, in the strict sense, refers to the motor integration used to execute complex learned movements. The reproduction of line drawings or block designs involves more than the organization of skilled hand movements. Such reproduction requires accurate visual perception, integration of perception into kinesthetic images, and translation of kinesthetic images into the final motor patterns that are necessary to produce the construction. Patients do not have to recognize or name the figure; they only have to develop an accurate concept or gestalt. The relations of angles and sides, the integration of parts into a whole, orientation on the page, and three-dimensionality must all be appreciated if accurate motor integration is to be carried out. The final step, of course, requires adequate limb strength and coordination.

Constructional impairment, rather than constructional apraxia, will be used to describe the failure to perform adequately on any of these tasks. As implied in the preceding paragraph, a disturbance in praxis (apraxia) refers only to a breakdown in the execution of the learned movements that are involved in the constructional task.[9] The term "apraxia" excludes the component of visual perception and organization and thus does not accurately describe the neuropsychologic complexity of the entire process.

EVALUATION

Constructional ability may be tested in a variety of ways, and different levels of performance may be found in the same patient when different tests are employed. To show the range of test materials that may be used, Warrington[22] has listed the following six basic types of tests for eliciting evidence of constructional impairment: (1) two-dimensional block designs, (2) paper-and-pencil reproduction of geometric shapes, (3) spontaneous drawings, (4) stick-pattern reproduction, (5) three-dimensional block constructions, and (6) spatial analysis tasks that require the patient to shade in the portion of a design that is common to two or more overlapping figures. Patients with brain lesions show differences in the incidence, severity, and quality of constructional impairment, depending on the type of test used and the nature and location of their lesions.[1,3,19]

The clinical examination of constructional impairment in the individual patient ideally should include several tests to tap somewhat different aspects of constructional ability; however, drawings to command and reproduction drawings remain the most easily administered and interpreted tests.

The use of the tests outlined in this book presumes that the patient has adequate vision (at least 20/100, as objectively tested) and sufficient motor ability to use paper, pencil, and blocks effectively. Deficits in either motor or sensory channels can hinder performance, but such impairment does not reflect the disruption in the integrative higher cortical function these tests are designed to assess. A number of constructional tests that include a memory component are available.[4,10,18] Although the inclusion of the memory component does increase the sensitivity of constructional tests, it also raises serious problems in the interpretation of the test results. Deficits in drawings from memory may be due to memory or constructional problems, or to a combination of the two. We believe that memory is a sufficiently important variable that it should be specifically tested in isolation. As we have emphasized throughout this book, a primary goal of each aspect of mental status testing is to assess as discrete a cognitive function as possible. The reader is referred to Appendix 1 for further information regarding the availability and description of visual memory tests.

The following brief tests of constructional ability are included for bed-side and office testing. These tests were chosen because of their ease of administration and interpretation, a limited need for apparatus and specialized equipment, and their proven efficacy in the detection of diffuse and focal brain lesions in patients with a wide range of intelligence.[21]

Reproduction Drawings

Directions: We suggest that reproduction drawings be administered first when assessing constructional ability because of their apparent simplicity and familiarity. The drawings presented in Figure 7–1 have been shown to be reproduced adequately by normal individuals, as well as being very sensitive to the effects of brain disease. They are organized in order of increasing difficulty and should be so administered. Both two- and three-dimensional drawings are used because of frequent quantitative and qualitative performance differences noted on these two somewhat different tasks. The examiner either may use a standard predrawn set of designs (probably best because the stimuli are identical for each administration and are generally of better quality than quickly drawn bedside examples) or may draw the stimulus figures on the left side of a piece of blank white paper. Separate sheets of paper for each design may be needed for patients who are highly distractible or perseverative. Lined progress-note forms, consult sheets, and other handy, but perceptually confusing, paper should not be used. It is often helpful to use two colors of pencil or felt-tip pen to reduce the possibility of confusion between the drawings of the patient and those drawn by a hurried examiner. Patients who become frustrated with their efforts on one drawing should be encouraged by the examiner to either start over or go on to the next drawing.

Introduce each item by saying, "Please draw this design exactly as it looks to you" (Fig. 7–1).

Scoring: To aid the examiner in quantifying the adequacy of patients' performance on this test, an objective scoring system[15] is provided for rating the relative quality of each drawing.

0—Poor	Given for nonrecognizable reproductions or a gross distortion of the basic design gestalt
1—Fair	Given for moderately distorted or rotated two-dimensional drawings or a loss of all three-dimensionality with moderate distortions or rotations on three-dimensional designs
2—Good	Given for minimal distortions or rotations with adequate integration on two-dimensional designs and some evidence of three-dimensionality but less-than-perfect reproduction on three-dimensional designs

Vertical Diamond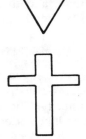

Two-Dimensional Cross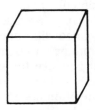

Three-Dimensional Block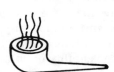

Three-Dimensional Pipe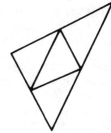

Triangle within a Triangle

Figure 7–1. Test items for Reproduction Drawings Test.

   3—Excellent   Given for perfect (or nearly perfect) reproductions of
                 two- and three-dimensional drawings

   Drawings that show evidence of rotations of more than 90 degrees
(Fig. 7–2, example 1); perseveration (Fig. 7–2, example 2); or "closing in"
(Fig. 7–2, example 3) are given ratings of 0.

Example 1 ROTATION

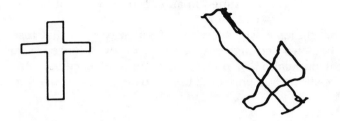

Example 2 PERSEVERATION

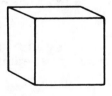

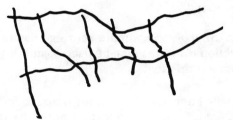

Example 3 "Closing In"

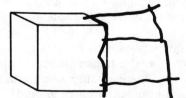

Figure 7–2. Examples of patient drawings with specific types of errors.

Standardization of these designs with nonselected brain-damaged and low-IQ (<80) normal people has indicated highly significant (P <.0001) differences in performance by the two groups on each design. A rating of 0 on any design resulted in a 100% probability of the patient being correctly classified as brain damaged, with a 0% probability of misclassification (false-positive). A rating of 1 resulted in an 80% probability of brain damage.[21]

Although the clinician will soon gain familiarity with this test and develop his or her own scoring criteria based on experience, examples from our clinical population of poor, fair, good, and excellent drawing reproductions are shown in Figures 7–3 to 7–7 to aid the examiner in rating each design.

Drawings to Command

Directions: The patient is required to draw three pictures to verbal command. Introduce the test by saying "I would now like you to draw some simple pictures on this paper. Draw each picture as well as you are able. Please draw a picture of a clock with the numbers and hands on it; a daisy in a flowerpot; a house in perspective so that you can see two sides and the roof."

Scoring: A simple scoring system similar to that used with reproduction drawings may be used to aid the examiner in quantifying performance on this test.

0—Poor	Given for nonrecognizable drawings or a gross distortion of the basic gestalt
1—Fair	Given for moderate distortion or rotation of any of the drawings or a loss of three-dimensionality on the house drawing (the clock should contain an approximately circular face or the numbers 1 through 12; the daisy should be recognizable as a flower in a pot; and the house should be recognizable as a house)
2—Good	Given for only mild distortions with adequate integration on all pictures (the house should contain some evidence of three-dimensionality and contain the basic elements of a house; the clock should contain two of the following: circular face, numbers 1 through 12, and symmetric number placement; the daisy should be in the generally appropriate shape—a circular center with petals around it)

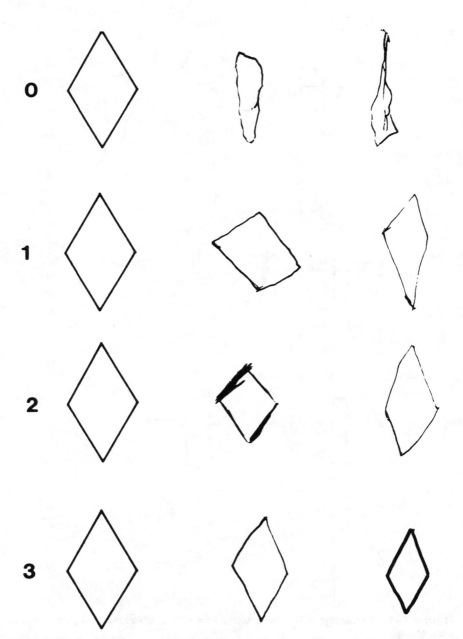

Figure 7–3. Renderings of Vertical Diamond Test, with scores of 0 (poor) through 3 (excellent).

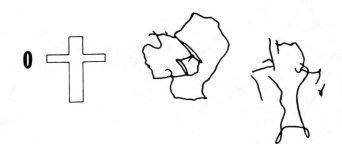

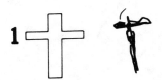

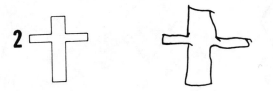

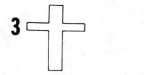

Figure 7–4. Renderings of Two-Dimensional Cross Test, with scores of 0 (poor) through 3 (excellent).

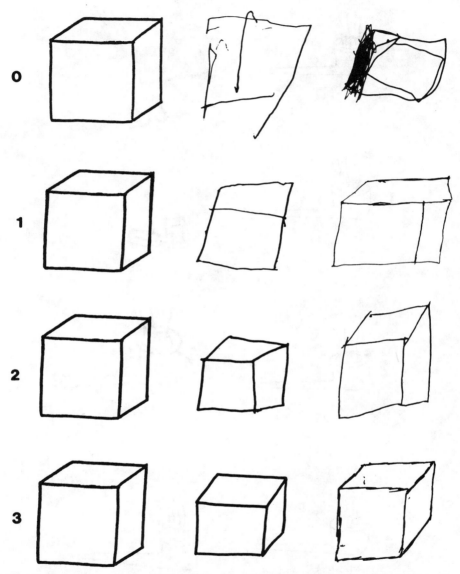

Figure 7–5. Renderings of Three-Dimensional Cube Test, with scores of 0 (poor) through 3 (excellent).

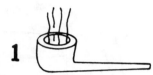
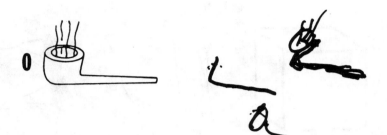
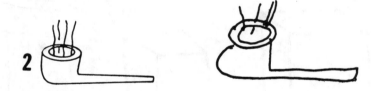

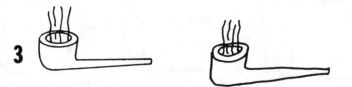

Figure 7–6. Renderings of Three-Dimensional Pipe Test, with scores of 0 (poor) through 3 (excellent).

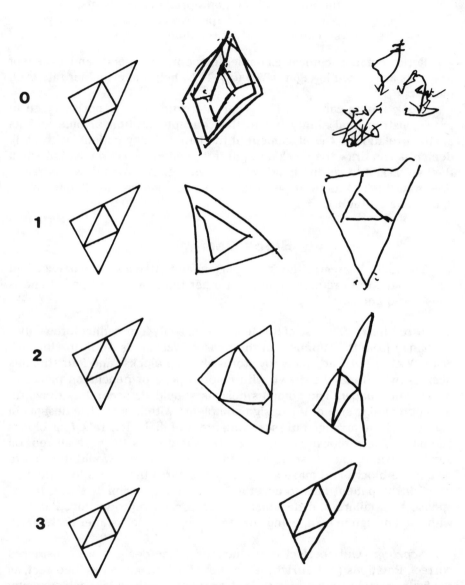

Figure 7–7. Renderings of triangle within a Triangle Test, with scores of 0 (poor) through 3 (excellent).

3—Excellent   Given for perfect (or near perfect) representations of the items with all appropriate components, placement, and perspective (the house and flowerpot should be clearly three-dimensional)

Representative clinical examples of poor, fair, good, and excellent drawings are shown in Figures 7–8 to 7–10 to help the examiner rate each picture.

Clock setting can often bring out interesting errors, not so much in pure constructional ability but in the conceptualization of time and its abstract relation to the placement of the hands. Many patients with early dementia can draw the clock and put in the numbers correctly, but when they are asked to set the hands at 2:30, will ponder, then draw a straight line from the 2 to the 6 or put in three hands (one on the 12, one on the 3, and one on the 6).

Block Designs

The following test, although important and often a source of excellent clinical data, does require equipment other than paper and pencil and is considered ancillary.

Directions: The use of this test requires only four multicolored cubes (obtained from the suppliers of the revised Wechsler's Adult Intelligence Scale [WAIS-R] or from many toy stores as Kohs blocks) and four stimulus designs, which may be drawn with colored pens or pencils on pieces of heavy white paper. The stimulus designs should be accurately drawn in the approximate size of the design completed with blocks. The designs in Figure 7–11 are arranged in ascending order of difficulty. Take four blocks and say, "These blocks are all alike. On some sides they are all red; on some, all white; and on some half red and half white. I would like you to take these blocks and make a design (or picture) that looks like this picture." If the patient fails to accurately reproduce design 1, score the response as a failure and demonstrate the correct reproduction. Continue with each design in turn, being sure to mix up the blocks after each effort.

Scoring: Only perfect reproductions of the designs are considered correct. Rotations (either right-left or near-far) are scored as incorrect, as are figure-ground (color) reversals. A score of 1 is given for each correctly reproduced design. Perfect reproductions of each design are expected from the normal individual.

Examples of commonly seen rotation, reversal, and "stringing out" errors are shown in Figure 7–12.

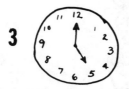

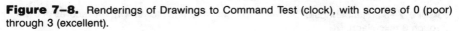

Figure 7–8. Renderings of Drawings to Command Test (clock), with scores of 0 (poor) through 3 (excellent).

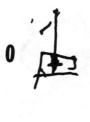

0

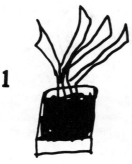

1

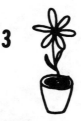

2

3

Figure 7–9. Renderings of Drawings to Command Test (flowerpot), with scores of 0 (poor) through 3 (excellent).

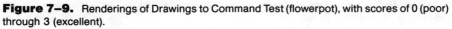

0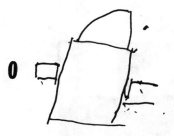

1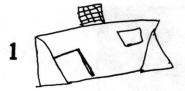

2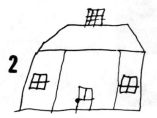

3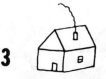

Figure 7–10. Renderings of Drawings to Command Test (house in perspective), with scores of 0 (poor) through 3 (excellent).

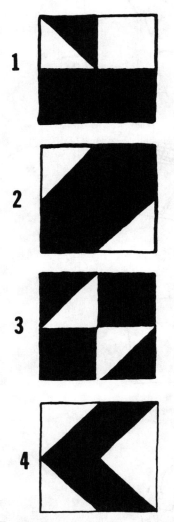

Figure 7–11. Test items for Block Designs Test.

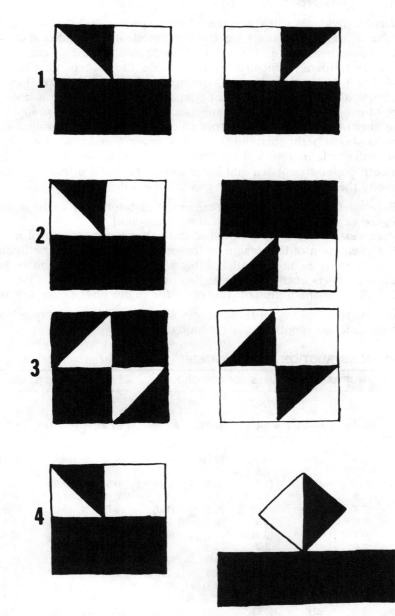

Figure 7–12. Examples of common errors on Block Designs Test. (1) Right-left rotation. (2) Near-far rotation. (3) Figure-ground reversal. (4) "Stringing out."

Interpreting Test Performance

Normal individuals will score almost perfect scores on simple reproduction and command drawings, but there is a modest yet significant drop-off in performance with age (Table 7–1). The three-dimensional cube and the house are the most difficult for most people. Close inspection of the data in Table 7–1 shows how much overlap there is among normal individuals, particularly the elderly and patients with early dementia. Subtle evidence of constructional impairment must be cautiously interpreted.

A number of specific types of errors on constructional tests are usually accepted as almost pathognomonic of brain damage when made by a non-retarded patient older than age 10. The majority of these errors can be seen on both paper-and-pencil and block-design tests. Of primary importance among these pathognomonic signs are the following:

1. Rotation by more than 45 degrees or the disorientation of the whole figure or a component of it on the background
2. Perseveration or the repetition of the entire figure or part of it
3. Fragmentation of the design or the omission of parts of the figure
4. Significant difficulty in either integration or the placement of individual parts at the correct angles or location
5. Substitution or addition of "dog ears" for angles on the drawn figure

The occurrence of any of these errors should raise a strong question of brain dysfunction requiring more detailed evaluation.

Table 7–1. CONSTRUCTION PERFORMANCE*

| | NORMAL INDIVIDUALS (BY AGE GROUP) | | | | | ALZHEIMER'S STAGE | | |
| | | | | | | I 71.3 (±7.8) | II 71.6 (±7.1) | III 71.5 (±8.9) |
	40–49	50–59	60–69	70–79	80–89			
Diamond	2.8	2.9	2.7	2.6	2.8	2.5	2.4	1.5
	(0.4)	(0.3)	(0.5)	(0.5)	(0.4)	(0.5)	(0.7)	(1.1)
Cross	2.8	2.8	2.6	2.2	2.2	2.2	1.9	1.2
	(0.4)	(0.4)	(0.5)	(0.5)	(0.6)	(0.9)	(0.8)	(1.0)
Cube	2.3	2.4	2.1	1.6	1.9	2.0	1.6	0.9
	(0.7)	(0.5)	(1.0)	(0.7)	(1.0)	(0.7)	(0.9)	(0.9)
Pipe	2.6	2.6	2.5	2.1	2.0	2.2	1.8	0.9
	(0.5)	(0.5)	(0.7)	(0.7)	(0.8)	(0.5)	(0.7)	(0.8)
Triangles	2.9	2.9	2.7	2.5	2.5	2.4	2.0	1.1
	(0.4)	(0.4)	(0.5)	(0.8)	(0.5)	(0.6)	(0.9)	(1.0)
Clock	2.9	3.0	2.5	2.3	2.1	2.7	1.8	0.6
	(0.3)	(0.2)	(0.7)	(0.7)	(0.9)	(0.5)	(1.0)	(0.9)
Flower	2.6	2.7	2.5	2.2	1.9	1.9	1.5	0.4
	(0.6)	(0.6)	(0.7)	(0.7)	(0.9)	(0.9)	(0.8)	(0.6)
House	2.2	2.5	2.2	2.1	1.9	1.8	1.4	0.5
	(0.7)	(0.5)	(0.7)	(0.7)	(0.8)	(0.9)	(0.9)	(0.8)

*Mean ±SD, on a scale of 0 to 3.

ANATOMY

The parietal lobes are the principal cortical areas involved in visuo-motor integration. The visual receptive areas of the occipital lobes and the motor areas of the frontal lobes are necessary for the completion of all of the tests, but it is the association cortex of the parietal lobes that is responsible for the complex integration. The actual localization of the various aspects of construction within the parietal lobes is not established, but it is postulated that visual stimuli are spread from primary sensory area 17 to contiguous secondary association areas of the inferior parietal lobule (areas 39 and 40), where associations are made between visual, auditory, and kinesthetic images.[16] Kinesthetic analysis of the visual pattern is the initial task of the association area. The kinesthetic images are then translated into motor patterns by involving the perirolandic premotor area. Drawings to command also require input from the auditory system. The premotor frontal association cortex would theoretically seem to be very important in these highly skilled, fine motor tasks, but, in fact, only a small percentage of patients with lesions restricted to the frontal lobes have constructional impairment.[7] The parietal lobes seem to be the major areas involved in learning and programming skilled movements; the frontal motor areas appear to be more involved in the pure executive nature of the task. (A more extensive discussion of learned skilled movements is in the section on apraxia in Chapter 9.)

CLINICAL IMPLICATIONS

If a nonretarded adult demonstrates constructional impairment on the tests outlined in this chapter, parietal lobe dysfunction can be strongly suspected. Although lesions in any quadrant of the brain can disrupt constructional performance, the incidence and severity of the deficits in patients with lesions that are restricted to the frontal lobes are small. Most constructional impairment is seen in patients with cortical damage posterior to the rolandic fissure.[7,13]

At one time, it was believed that the right (nondominant) parietal lobe was actually dominant for constructional ability. Many studies have been performed comparing the relative incidence and severity of constructional impairment in patients with lesions of the right and left hemispheres. These studies clearly demonstrate that performance can be defective with lesions in either parietal lobe.[17] In general, right hemisphere lesions produce a higher incidence and greater severity of defect than do left hemisphere lesions.[3] What is certain is that constructional ability is not a function exclusive to the right parietal lobe.[11]

Some subtle differences in qualitative performance that are both interesting and possibly useful in clinical testing have been noted in patients with right and left parietal lobe lesions. On the block designs test, patients with right hemisphere lesions frequently lose the basic outline of the design and "string out" the blocks.[12] This is shown in example 4, Figure 7–12. These patients tend to make scattered and fragmented drawings that show loss of spatial relations and orientation on the page. Patients with left hemisphere lesions show more coherent block designs, with maintenance of external configuration but loss of accurate internal detail (example 3, Fig. 7–12). Their drawings tend to be simplifications of the model, lacking detail but having preserved general spatial relationships. Obvious differences in the performance of the two groups are not always seen, and elaborate scoring schemes have been designed to bring out the subtle differences.[5] Such systems are interesting but are probably not of practical significance to the bedside clinician. The quality of constructional impairment with right hemisphere lesions is uniform and will not differ according to the locus of the lesion within the hemisphere.[14] Without very careful assessment of qualitative performance and using constructional tests alone, it is not always possible to determine the side of the lesion in the individual patient unless unilateral neglect is present. When a patient's constructional ability is grossly impaired, in the face of normal language, right hemisphere dysfunction is strongly suggested.

Patients with lesions that are confined to the parietal lobes will often show evidence of significant constructional impairment on mental status testing yet will fail to demonstrate abnormalities on the standard neurologic examination. Therefore, the presence of errors on constructional testing should lead to a more complete neurodiagnostic workup.

The most dramatic examples of constructional impairment occur in patients with bilateral cortical disease. This is particularly well demonstrated in cerebral atrophy. Patients with Alzheimer's disease (by far the most common dementia) can show constructional difficulty in the early stages of their disease (Table 7–1).[20] The patients with multiple infarct dementia, seen in cerebral vascular disease, may also show constructional impairment, but they usually have other abnormal neurologic signs as well. Patients in confusional states from toxic or metabolic factors frequently demonstrate constructional impairment during the acute stage. This is secondary to reversible physiologic disturbance of the cortex rather than to structural damage.

Because of the fairly high incidence of constructional impairment in dementia, such tasks are very good screening tests in patients of advancing age who present with vague psychiatric or neurologic complaints.

Standard drawing and other constructional tests are used not only to detect brain disease, but also by psychologists to evaluate both the maturational stage of perceptuomotor development (constructional ability) and the presence of specific constructional problems in children. The ability to integrate visual stimuli and to construct or draw a reproduction is closely related to both chronologic and intellectual maturation in young children.[2,8,15] Errors in construction, including poor integration of the parts, distortions or simplification, perseveration, and rotations, are common early in development (age 5 to 7 years) and tend to decrease with age.[6] Relatively errorless performance on simple drawing tests is expected by age 10 to 12.[15] Measured intelligence tends to be relatively highly correlated with constructional performance in children; for adults of normal intelligence (i.e., IQ above 85) IQ appears to have a limited effect on constructional ability.[18] Both children and adults with a significant mental deficiency tend to show inferior performance on most constructional tests.[4] Formal studies have indicated that it is difficult but not impossible to use drawing tests to differentiate intellectually impaired (e.g., IQ below 70) but socially and vocationally independent adults from similar individuals with demonstrable brain damage.[21]

As with any skilled motor activity, both initial exposure and repeated practice affect the ability to reproduce paper-and-pencil designs or to complete block constructions. Social deprivation and a lack of academic experience do, therefore, have a detrimental effect on constructional performance. Therefore, the clinician who uses constructional tests as a part of the mental status examination must be cautious in interpreting the results of performance of patients with a history of retardation or a poor academic background, or both. Placed in the proper interpretive context, however, drawings and other constructional tests may be fruitfully used with such patients.

SUMMARY

Constructional ability is a highly developed cortical integrative function that is primarily carried out in the parietal lobes. Drawings and block constructions are easily administered tests to evaluate this function. Impairment of constructional performance usually suggests disease of the posterior portions of the cerebral hemispheres, although other areas of the cortex may be involved. Because constructional ability is so frequently disturbed in patients with brain disease, testing this function is a very important and highly useful component of the mental status examination.

REFERENCES

1. Arrigoni, G and De Renzi, E: Constructional apraxia and hemispheric locus of lesions. Cortex 1:170, 1964.
2. Bender, L: A Visual Motor Gestalt Test and its Clinical Use. American Orthopsychiatric Association, New York, 1938.
3. Benson, DF and Barton, M: Disturbances in constructional ability. Cortex 6:19, 1970.
4. Benton, A: Revised Visual Retention Test. The Psychological Corporation, New York, 1974.
5. Benton, AL: Visuoperceptive, visuospatial and visuoconstructive disorders. In Heilman, KM and Valenstein, E (eds): Clinical Neuropsychology. Oxford University Press, New York, 1979, pp 186–232.

6. Black, FW: Reversal and rotation errors by normal and retarded readers. Percept Mot Skills 36:895, 1973.
7. Black, FW and Strub, RL: Constructional apraxia in patients with discrete missile wounds of the brain. Cortex 12:212, 1976.
8. Frostig, M, Lefever, D and Whittlesey, J: A developmental test of visual perception for evaluating normal and neurologically handicapped children. Percept Mot Skills 12:383, 1961.
9. Geschwind, N: The apraxias: neural mechanisms of disorders of learned movement. Am Sci 63:188, 1975.
10. Graham, F and Kendall, B: Memory for Designs Test. Psychology Test Specialists, Missoula, Mont., 1960.
11. Hécaen, H: Apraxias. In Filskov, SB and Boll, TJ (eds): Handbook of Clinical Neuropsychology. John Wiley & Sons, New York, 1981, pp 267–286.
12. Kaplan, E: Personal communication, 1973.
13. Kertesz, A: Right hemisphere lesions in constructional apraxia and visuospatial deficit. In Kertesz, A (ed): Localization in Neuropsychology. Academic Press, New York, 1983, pp 455–570.
14. Kertesz, A and Dobrowski, S: Right hemisphere deficits, lesion size and location. J Clin Neuropsychol 3:283, 1981.
15. Koppitz, E: The Bender Gestalt Test for Young Children. Grune & Stratton, New York, 1964.
16. Luria, A: The Working Brain. Basic Books, New York, 1973.
17. Mack, JL and Levine, RN: The basis of visual constructional disability in patients with unilateral cerebral lesions. Cortex 17:515, 1981.
18. Pascal, G and Suttell, B: The Bender Gestalt Test. Grune & Stratton, New York, 1951.
19. Piercy, M, Hécaen, H, and De Ajuriaguerra, J: Constructional apraxia associated with unilateral lesions: Left and right cases compared. Brain 83:232, 1960.
20. Sjörgen, T, Sjörgen, T, and Lindgren, AGH: Mörbus Alzheimer and Mörbus Pick: A genetic, clinical, and pathoanatomical study. Acta Psychiatr Scand (Suppl)82:1, 1952.
21. Strub, RL, Black, FW, and Leventhal, B: The clinical utility of reproduction drawings with low IQ patients. J Clin Psychiatry 40:386, 1979.
22. Warrington, E: Constructional apraxia. In Vinken, P and Bruyn, G (eds): Handbook of Clinical Neurology, Vol 4, Disorders of Speech, Perception and Symbolic Behavior. American Elsevier, Amsterdam, 1969, pp 67–83.

Chapter 8

Higher Cognitive Functions

Attention, language, and memory are the basic processes that serve as building blocks for the development of higher intellectual abilities. These basic functions are necessary, but not sufficient in and of themselves, to execute more complex cognitive functions. "Higher cognitive functions" refers to the highest level of human intellectual functioning readily assessable by formal testing methods. Included within this category of functions are the manipulation of well-learned material, abstract thinking, problem-solving, arithmetic computations, and so forth. These complex neuropsychologic functions are predicated on the integrity and interaction of more basic processes.

Because they represent the most advanced stages of intellectual development, the higher cognitive functions are often highly susceptible to the effects of neurologic disease. The evaluation of these functions in the mental status examination may often demonstrate the early effects of cortical damage before the more basic processes of attention, language, and memory are impaired. The ability to perform effectively within the environment is determined in large part by an individual's adequacy in performing such higher-order functions. An assessment of the patient's performance in these areas will provide useful diagnostic information, as well as information concerning social and vocational prognosis.

EVALUATION

There are many different ways to evaluate the higher cognitive functions; most intelligence tests are largely based on assessments of these functions. In general, the higher cognitive functions may be categorized in the following hierarchic groupings: (1) the fund of acquired information or the store of knowledge; (2) the manipulation of old knowledge (e.g., calculations or problem solving); (3) social awareness and judgment; and (4) abstract thinking (e.g., the interpretation of proverbs or the completion of a conceptual series). The store of basic acquired information is most efficiently assessed by simple verbal tests of vocabulary, general information, and comprehension. Specific examples of these kinds of tests may be seen on any basic intelligence test (e.g., revised Wechsler's Adult Intelligence Scale [WAIS-R] Vocabulary, Information, Picture Completion). General intelligence, education, and social exposure are closely related to performance on these tasks, and the results of any evaluation must be interpreted in light of this background information.

The manipulation of old knowledge is a more active process, which involves both an intact fund of general information and the ability to apply this information to new or unfamiliar situations. Questions concerning social comprehension and calculation ability may be used to assess this function. Social awareness and problem solving may be evaluated by questions concerning the knowledge of environmental situations and how to deal with them effectively (e.g., What should a person do if he or she sees smoke or fire in a grocery store?).

Social judgment is a more complex function that includes the basic knowledge of social situations, the socially appropriate response in such situations, and the ability to personally apply the correct response when faced with a genuine situation. Because of the reality-based nature of social judgment, it is difficult to assess validly in an abstract test situation. The patient who matter-of-factly states that he or she would calmly inform the manager of the presence of smoke or fire in the store when asked the question in the confines of an office or hospital bed may act very differently when faced with the actual situation. Therefore, collaborative data concerning the patient's social judgment are best obtained by history from family or other informants who have witnessed the patient's actual performance in dealing with day-to-day events. An alternative possibility, albeit a somewhat cumbersome and inefficient procedure, is to place the patient in actual, but experimental, situations that require an immediate, appropriate social response.

Abstract thinking, which is perhaps the highest level of cognition, may be readily assessed by the use of proverbs, conceptual series, or analogy interpretation.

The following tests are recommended to evaluate a spectrum of relevant higher cognitive functions.

Fund of Information

Directions: The following questions provide a reasonable estimate of the patient's store of knowledge or fund of general information. They are presented in order of increasing difficulty and should be so administered. If it is obvious from the history or interview that the patient is of above-average intelligence, some of the less difficult questions may be omitted. Continue to ask questions until the test is completed or until the patient has failed three successive questions. If the patient's response is unclear, ask him or her to explain more fully. The examiner may repeat the question if necessary but should not paraphrase the question or spell or explain words that are unfamiliar to the patient.

TEST ITEMS

QUESTIONS	ACCEPTABLE RESPONSES
1. How many weeks are in a year?	52
2. Why do people have lungs?	To transfer oxygen from air to blood; to breath
3. Name four people who have been president of the United States since 1940.	Any appropriate presidents
4. Where is Denmark?	Scandinavia, Northern Europe
5. How far is it from New York to Los Angeles?	Any answer between 2300 and 3000 miles.
6. Why are light-colored clothes cooler in the summer than dark-colored clothes?	Light-colored clothes reflect heat from the sun whereas dark-colored clothes absorb heat
7. What is the capital of Spain?	Madrid
8. What causes rust?	Oxidation: a chemical reaction of metal, oxygen, and moisture
9. Who wrote the Odyssey?	Homer
10. What is the Acropolis?	Site of the Parthenon in Athens, Greece; ancient city on a hill in Athens

Scoring: The acceptable response for each question is provided. The patient's answer must either be exact or very closely approximate the acceptable response. In our experience, the average patient with an adequate educational background should answer a minimum of six questions appropriately (Table 8–1). The fund of information is quite stable over a wide age range; only in the 80s does one find a small yet statistically significant dropoff in this function. By contrast, patients with Alzheimer's disease—even those with mild disease—score only an average of 3.5 of a possible 10 on this task. Less adequate performance indicates an impaired

Table 8–1. FUND OF INFORMATION TEST*

NORMAL INDIVIDUALS (BY AGE GROUP)					PATIENTS WITH ALZHEIMER'S DISEASE (BY STAGE)			
40–49	50–59	60–69	70–79	80–89	I	II	III	IV
6.7 (2.5)	6.8 (1.9)	6.5 (2.0)	6.3 (2.0)	5.2 (1.5)	3.5 (3.9)	2.0 (2.9)	0.6 (1.1)	0 (0)

*Mean number correct (± SD).

fund of general information and is suspicious of retardation, limited social and educational exposure, or significant dementia. Conversely, more adequate performance suggests above-average intelligence and education.

Calculations

Directions: Calculations are complex neuropsychologic functions that involve the somewhat distinct components of (1) rote tables (e.g., addition, subtraction, and multiplication); (2) the basic arithmetic concept of carrying and borrowing; (3) recognition of the signs ($+$, $-$, $\times$, $\div$); and (4) correct spatial alignment for written calculations.[8] Because these components of calculations may be disturbed in isolation, they are assessed separately in this section. When evaluating calculations, it is important to require the patient actually to calculate and not merely to recite rote tables (e.g., $4 + 4 = 8$ or $3 \times 5 = 15$). This allows the observation of many different types of errors and provides additional clinical data that are important for a description of the nature of the deficit and for providing neuroanatomic implications. Performance on calculation is, of course, closely related to educational experience. Tell the patient, "We are now going to do some arithmetic examples. Some will be familiar to you and some will not. Try your best on each one."

Verbal Rote Examples

Read each example in a clear voice in the following form: "What is 4 plus 6?" Record the patient's response.

1. Addition
   $4 + 6 = (10)$
   $7 + 9 = (16)$

2. Subtraction
   $8 - 5 = (3)$
   $17 - 9 = (8)$

3. Multiplication
   $2 \times 8 = (16)$
   $9 \times 7 = (63)$

4. Division
   $9 \div 3 = (3)$
   $56 \div 8 = (7)$

Verbal Complex Examples

Read each example in the following form only once: "What is 8 plus 13?" Allow only 20 seconds for a response; a failure to respond within that time, even if a correct response is ultimately given, is scored as a failure. Record the patient's response.

1. Addition
   $14 + 17 = (31)$

2. Subtraction
   $43 - 38 = (5)$

3. Multiplication
   $21 \times 5 = (105)$

4. Division
   $128 \div 8 = (16)$

Written Complex Examples

Provide the patient with the following written examples. If the patient is inattentive and distractible, it is useful to provide each example on individual cards or to write each new example after the patient completes the previous example. Examples written on a single sheet of paper should be widely separated. Allow a reasonable amount of time for completion of each example. Failure to complete the example within 30 seconds should be noted. Record the patient's response, including errors in alignment.

1. Addition
   108
   $+ 79$

2. Subtraction
   605
   $- 86$

3. Multiplication
   108
   $\times 36$

4. Division
   43$\overline{)559}$

Scoring: Each response should be scored as correct or incorrect. By comparing performance on each computation subtest, the patient's overall level of calculation ability and area of adequacy and deficit can be determined (e.g., intact rote tables, with inability to complete complex, verbally presented examples). Errors specific to a particular aspect of computation (e.g., division) or to a modality of presentation (e.g., intact performance on verbally presented items and impaired performance on written examples) should be noted. Errors involving borrowing and alignment on written examples should be recorded (Fig. 8–1). If an objective measure of arithmetic is needed, the examiner should refer to a standard achievement test such as the Wide Range Achievement Test–Revised.[7] Calculation ability is stable across all age groups, although variable performance is seen within each group (Table 8–2). Performance in early dementia is not significantly impaired, particularly in the older patients. Performance deteriorates dramatically in the second and third stages of the disease.

Proverb Interpretation

Directions: Interpreting proverbs accurately requires an intact fund of general information, the ability to apply this knowledge to unfamiliar situations, and the ability to think in the abstract. The following proverbs are presented in ascending order of difficulty. Tell the patient, "I am going to read you a saying that you may or may not have heard before. Explain in your own words what the saying means." Read each proverb exactly as written. Do not paraphrase or otherwise explain the proverb. Continue only until the patient fails on two successive proverbs. If the patient's response to the first proverb is concrete (nonabstract), or if he or she is unable to

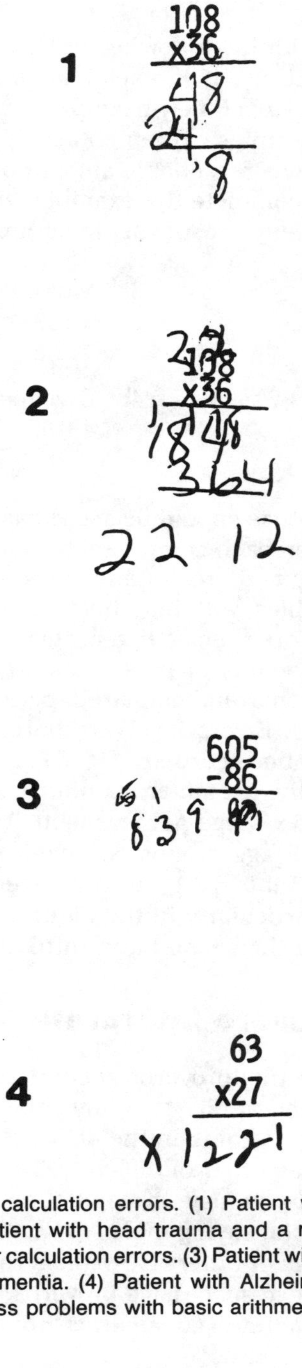

1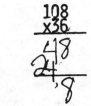

2

3

4

Figure 8–1. Examples of calculation errors. (1) Patient with a large right-hemisphere lesion and left neglect. (2) Patient with head trauma and a right parietal hematoma. Note poor alignment as well as other calculation errors. (3) Patient with 2 years of college education now shows signs of early dementia. (4) Patient with Alzheimer's disease. Note that rote multiplication is good, but gross problems with basic arithmetic processes exist.

Table 8-2. TESTS OF CALCULATION ABILITY*

	NORMAL INDIVIDUALS (BY AGE GROUP)					PATIENTS WITH ALZHEIMER'S DISEASE (BY STAGE)			
	40-49	50-59	60-69	70-79	80-89	I	II	III	IV
Verbal	3.7	3.7	3.7	3.4	3.7	3.6	3.1	1.6	0
rote	(0.7)	(0.6)	(0.7)	(1.0)	(0.5)	(0.6)	(1.0)	(1.6)	0
Verbal	2.9	3.1	3.2	2.4	2.9	2.9	1.2	0.3	0
complex	(1.3)	(0.9)	(0.8)	(1.3)	(1.4)	(1.3)	(1.3)	(0.8)	0
Written	3.4	3.2	3.4	2.8	3.2	2.7	1.9	0.4	0
	(1.3)	(1.1)	(0.6)	(1.3)	(0.8)	(1.0)	(1.2)	(0.8)	0

*Mean number correct (±SD).

interpret it, the examiner should supply the correct answer and explain that this is the expected type of response.

Test Items
1. Don't cry over spilled milk.
2. Rome wasn't built in a day.
3. A drowning man will clutch at a straw.
4. A golden hammer breaks an iron door.
5. The hot coal burns; the cold one blackens.

Scoring: The primary scoring criterion for proverb interpretation is the degree of abstraction demonstrated by the patient in explaining the proverb. It is helpful to rate the quality of the patient's response to each proverb. To aid the examiner, examples of abstract (2 points); semiabstract (1 point); and concrete (0 points) responses to each proverb are provided below. Total for this section is 10 points.

1. Don't cry over spilled milk
   0—Concrete   "The milk's all over the floor."
                   "When the milk is on the floor, you can't use it."
   1—Semiabstract "It's gone; don't worry about it."
                   "Don't cry when something goes wrong."
   2—Abstract   "Once something is over, don't worry about it."
                   "Don't be concerned about events that are beyond control."

2. Rome wasn't built in a day.
   0—Concrete   "It took a long time to build Rome."
                   "You can't build cities overnight."
   1—Semiabstract "Don't do things too fast."
                   "You have to be patient and careful."

  2—Abstract   "If something is worth doing, it is worth doing
                        it carefully."
                      "It takes time to do things well."

3. A drowning man will clutch at a straw.
   0—Concrete   "Don't let go when you're in the water."
                      "He's trying to save himself."
   1—Semiabstract   "Self-preservation is important."
                      "It's a last resort."
   2—Abstract   "A person in trouble will try anything to get
                        out of it."
                      "If sufficiently desperate, a person will try
                        anything."

4. A golden hammer breaks an iron door.
   0—Concrete   "Gold can't break iron!"
                      "Gold is too soft to break a door."
   1—Semiabstract   "Gold's worth more than iron."
                      "The harder something is, the more you have
                        to work to get it."
   2—Abstract   "Virtue conquers all."
                      "If you have sufficient knowledge, you can
                        accomplish even the most difficult task."

5. The hot coal burns; the cold one blackens.
   0—Concrete   "Hot coals will burn you and leave it black."
                      "Hot coals get black when they're cold."
   1—Semiabstract   "Coal can have many uses."
                      "Getting burned and dirty are both bad."
   2—Abstract   "Extremes of anything can be detrimental."
                      "There may be bad aspects to things that
                        appear good."

Concrete responses are pathologic in all but the retarded or illiterate patient. The average patient should provide abstract interpretations to at least the first three proverbs and minimally semiabstract responses to the remaining proverbs. Often, uneducated patients will initially give a concrete response but can give abstract interpretations when specifically asked if there is another way of explaining the proverb. Such cued responses should be scored as a semiabstract response. A total score of less than 5 on proverb interpretation is suspicious. A concrete response or an absence of any abstract responses should suggest an impairment of abstract ability.

Performance on proverb interpretation is stable across all ages (Table 8–3). The high standard deviation within the normal population, however, shows how cautious the examiner must be in interpreting a low score on this task. Patients with early Alzheimer's disease score only slightly lower

Table 8–3. TESTS OF VERBAL ABSTRACTION*

NORMAL INDIVIDUALS (BY AGE GROUP)					PATIENTS WITH ALZHEIMER'S DISEASE (BY STAGE)			
40–49	50–59	60–69	70–79	80–89	I	II	III	IV
Proverbs								
5.1	5.1	4.4	4.3	5.6	4.0	1.8	0.5	0
(1.5)	(1.5)	(2.2)	(1.6)	(1.3)	(2.3)	(1.5)	(0.9)	(0)
Similarities								
6.0	5.9	5.0	4.5	5.1	4.9	2.8	0.9	0
(2.5)	(1.9)	(2.3)	(2.0)	(2.6)	(2.1)	(2.1)	(1.4)	(0)

*Mean score (± SD).

on an average than normal individuals do. As dementia progresses, performance drops rapidly. In general, a score of 2 or 3 on proverb interpretation in educated individuals is indicative of organic impairment.

Similarities

Directions: In the Verbal Similarities Test the patient must explain the basic similarity between two overtly different objects or situations. This test of verbal abstract ability requires analysis of relationships, formation of verbal concepts, and logical thinking. Tell the patient, "I am going to tell you some pairs of objects. Each pair is alike in some way. Please tell me how they are similar, or alike." If the patient mentions a difference between the items, fails to respond, or states that they are different, score the item 0, provide the appropriate response, and continue with the next item. Give no help on succeeding items. The following test items are presented in ascending order of difficulty.

TEST ITEMS
1. Turnip—Cauliflower
2. Car—Airplane
3. Desk—Bookcase
4. Poem—Novel
5. Horse—Apple

Scoring: The response for each item pair is scored for adequacy. Two points should be given for any abstract similarity or general classification that is highly pertinent for both items in the pair. One point should be given for responses that indicate specific properties of both items in the pair and that constitute a relevant similarity. A score of 0 is given when the response reflects properties of only one member of the pair, differences, generalizations that are not pertinent to the item pair, and failures to respond. Examples of responses receiving 2 points, 1 point, and 0 points are provided. Total for this section is 10 points.

1. Turnip—Cauliflower
   2 points: Vegetables
   1 point: Food; they grow in the ground; edible
   0 points: Buy in the store; one is a root, the other grows above ground

2. Car—Airplane
   2 points: Modes of transportation
   1 point: Drive them both, have motors
   0 points: One's in the air and one's on the road

3. Desk—Bookcase
   2 points: Articles of furniture
   1 point: Household objects; office furniture; put books on them, made of the same material
   0 points: Sit at a desk and put books in the bookcase, for studying

4. Poem—Novel
   2 points: Literary works or types of literature; artistic works; modes of creative expression
   1 point: Write them both; tell stories; express feelings
   0 points: Famous things; study them in school; people like them

5. Horse—Apple
   2 points: Living things; God's living objects, organic things
   1 point: Both grow; both have skins; both need food
   0 points: Horses eat apples; one is big and one is small; we use them

The nonretarded patient with a normal educational background should obtain a score of 5 or 6 on this test (Table 8–3). Two concrete (0-point) responses or a total score of less than 4 suggests reduced general intelligence or impaired abstract ability. In general, performance on this test should be compatible with performance on the test of fund of information and proverb interpretation. If similarities and fund of information test performances are equally impaired, this is suggestive of retardation or educational deprivation rather than a specific deficit in abstract thinking.

Conceptual Series Completion

Directions: The conceptual series completion is another test of verbal abstraction, the ability to solve unfamiliar and complex verbal problems, and the ability to reason at a high level. Tell the patient, "I am going to show you some numbers, letters, or words in series. Each series will be incomplete and needs an additional word, letter, or number to complete it. Each dash (−) calls for either a number or a letter to be filled in. Take each item in order, but if you don't understand it, don't spend too much time on any one item." The following sequences are presented to the patient in written form, either on a standard form prepared beforehand by the examiner or written on a sheet of paper by the examiner.

TEST ITEMS

SERIES	CORRECT RESPONSE
1. ABCD __	E
2. 1 4 7 10 __ __	13
3. AZ BY CX D __	W
4. tote to snow on spun up stab __ __	at
5. elephant 87654321 plan 5732 lap __ __ __	735

Scoring: Each response is scored as correct or incorrect using the foregoing scoring criteria. No unique or original interpretations of the correct response are allowed. Excellent performance (four or five correct) on this task certainly indicates a high degree of conceptual ability, but we have found that normal individuals average only two (80-year-olds) to three (40- to 70-year-olds) correct out of five. The standard deviation is high and therefore this item has not proved to be a very sensitive indicator of pathology, and we no longer use it.

ANATOMY

The higher cognitive functions rely primarily on an intact cerebral cortex. They are not, however, functions that have been well localized in the way that language or constructional ability has. Abstract thinking, the ability to manipulate old knowledge, calculation ability, and similar functions are probably widely represented in the cortex. Subcortical structures are also important in carrying out these highly abstract functions. Because of this diffuse representation, an impairment of these functions can result from lesions that are located in various parts of the brain. Impairment is particularly prominent in widespread bilateral disease (e.g., dementia).

It is likely that these higher cognitive functions are localized in the posterior rather than frontal areas of the brain. Although a loss of abstraction has been described in patients following frontal lobectomies[9] and has been traditionally considered a sign of extensive frontal lobe dysfunction, patients with frontal lobe damage have defects of attention, memory, and perseveration that may well account for the observed deficits in higher cognition.[6,10] In a comprehensive review of the literature concerned with the interaction of frontal lesions and cognitive functioning, Teuber[11] concluded that such lesions generally affect intelligence less than do lesions located in the more posterior areas of the brain. Black[1] also documented the differential effects of frontal and nonfrontal unilateral lesions on cognitive functions. This study again verified that these higher cognitive functions are more commonly impaired with posterior lesions.

Verbal reasoning and abstraction are primarily dominant hemisphere functions with very close relationships with language. Thus, dominant hemisphere lesions frequently interfere with these high-level verbal manipulations.

Impaired performance on calculations may be seen with brain lesions that are bilateral or unilateral on either the right or the left side.[4] Lesions in somewhat different areas of the brain may cause different types of impaired calculation ability (dyscalculia).[3] Left hemisphere lesions in the right-handed patient typically result in more severe impairment of calculations than do corresponding lesions of the nondominant hemisphere.[2] A significant dyscalculia often accompanies aphasia. Similarly, dyscalculia is a significant component of Gerstmann's syndrome (described in Chapter 9), which is secondary to a dominant parietal lobe lesion. Specific calculation defects ascribed to focal frontal, temporal, parietal, and occipital lesions have been described.[5] Impaired calculation ability due to focal lesions in the parietal lobes appears to be more common. This type of disorder is characterized by a loss of the ability to understand the meaning of numbers and numeric concepts (e.g., larger or smaller) and by the inability to align numbers correctly on the page owing to visual-spatial deficits. The malalignment in complex computations can often be the most striking feature in the dyscalculia seen in patients with parietal lobe lesions.

CLINICAL IMPLICATIONS

Deficits in higher cognitive functions are most frequently seen in patients with widespread brain disease of any etiology. These deficits may often be the first sign of deterioration in progressive brain diseases such as Alzheimer's disease. Focal dominant parietal lobe lesions may produce defects in verbally mediated functions and must be considered in the differential diagnosis in any patient presenting with a loss of abstract ability or impaired calculations. As discussed previously, lesions of the frontal lobe typically do not interfere with the fund of knowledge, abstract thinking, and problem solving unless other, more basic deficits are also present (e.g., perseveration or aphasia). Conversely, social awareness and judgment in social situations are often impaired in patients with large frontal lesions.

Significant functional disease, particularly schizophrenia, may cause impaired abstracting ability. Although the concreteness of the schizophrenic patient is frequently different from that of the patient with organic brain disease (e.g., symbolic interpretations incorporating the patient's delusions), at times the deficit may be indistinguishable from that seen in patients with organic disease.

Because of the close relationship between higher cognitive function and general intelligence, mental retardation from whatever cause will result in impaired performance on these tests. Educational deprivation will similarly result in substandard performance that is not of diagnostic significance. Accordingly, performance on the tests of higher cognitive function must be interpreted within the context of both educational background and premorbid intelligence. The test of fund of information provides a reasonable estimate of current intellectual functioning, which may be combined with data from the history to furnish this background information.

SUMMARY

Higher cognitive functions are measures of the patient's reasoning and problem-solving abilities. These functions are often impaired early in brain disease and thereby offer an effective measure for detecting brain disease in patients with relatively intact performance in other areas (e.g., language or constructional ability). Any deficits will be reflected in the patient's inability to function effectively within the environment. Thus, an evaluation of these functions will aid in making a valid social and vocational prognosis.

REFERENCES

1. Black, W: Cognitive deficits in patients with unilateral war-related frontal lobe lesions. J Clin Psychol 32:366, 1976.
2. Boller, F and Grafman, J: Acalculia: Historical development and current significance. Brain Cognition 2:205, 1983.
3. Ferro, JM and Botello, MAS: Alexia for arithmetical signs. A cause of disturbed calculations. Cortex 16:175, 1980.
4. Critchley, M: The Parietal Lobes. Edward Arnold, London, 1953.
5. Grewel, F: Acalculias. In Vinken, P and Bruyn, G (eds): Handbook of Clinical Neurology, Vol 4, Disorders of Speech, Perception, and Symbolic Behavior. American Elsevier, New York, 1969, pp 181–194.
6. Hécaen, H and Albert, M: Disorders of mental functioning related to frontal lobe pathology. In Benson, DF and Blumer, D (eds): Psychiatric Aspects of Neurologic Disease. Grune & Stratton, New York, 1975, pp 137–149.
7. Jastak, S and Wilkenson, GS: The Wide Range Achievement Test-Revised. Jastak Associates, Wilmington, DE, 1984.
8. Kahn, HJ (ed): Cognitive and Neuropsychological Aspects of Calculation Disorders. Brain Cognition 17:97, 1991 (special issue).
9. Rylander, G: Mental Changes After Excision of Cerebral Tissue. Ejnar Munksgaards Forlag, Copenhagen, 1943.
10. Stuss, DT and Benson, DF: Neuropsychological studies of the frontal lobes. Psychol Monogr 95:1, 1984.
11. Teuber, HL: The riddle of frontal lobe function in man. In Warren, J and Akert, K (eds): The Frontal Granular Cortex and Behavior. McGraw-Hill, New York, 1964, pp 410–444.

Chapter 9

Related Cortical Functions

Several specific disorders of cortical function have been of great interest to neurologists and neuropsychologists. Most are related to high-level motor and sensory processing. For instance, apraxia is an example of a high-level motor disturbance, and visual agnosia is a high-level perceptual disturbance. These disorders are of some utility in cerebral localization and are of considerable research interest to neurobehaviorists. Because each disorder is relatively discrete, a complete discussion of each disorder, including terminology, evaluation, and clinical implications, is presented.

APRAXIA

Apraxia is an acquired disorder of learned, sequential motor movements that cannot be accounted for by elementary disturbances of strength, coordination, sensation, or lack of comprehension or attention.[25] It is an impairment in selecting and organizing the motor innervations needed to execute an action.[3] Apraxia is not a low-level motor disturbance but rather a defect in motor planning, which involves the integrative steps that precede skilled or learned movements. Different types of apraxia have been described, based on the complexity and nature of the task performed.

A motor disturbance characterized by clumsiness or involuntary grasp reflexes in the limb contralateral to a cortical lesion[15] is called a limb-kinetic apraxia. Because patients with this disturbance have difficulty with basic motor control and display abnormal reflexes, their movements do not meet the classic requirements of apraxia.

Ideomotor Apraxia

Ideomotor apraxia is the most common type of apraxia. Patients having this form of apraxia fail to perform previously learned motor acts accurately. Impairment can be seen in buccofacial, upper or lower limb, or truncal musculature. The inability to carry out such commands as "Show me how you blow out a match" or "Drink through a straw" is called buccofacial apraxia. Difficulty with arm or leg movements such as flipping a coin, saluting, or kicking a ball is called limb apraxia. Difficulty with truncal commands such as "Curtsy," "Swing a baseball bat," or "Stand like a boxer" is called an apraxia of whole body movements.

Evaluation

There is a hierarchy of difficulty in performing these ideomotor tasks. The most difficult level requires the patient to perform the action to verbal command (e.g., "Show me how to flip a coin"). This movement must be mimed without the coin and without any nonverbal cues from the examiner. If the patient fails at this level, the examiner performs the action and asks the patient to imitate it. Imitation is easier for most patients with apraxia. If the patient again fails, provide the real object and again ask the patient to follow the command. Use of the actual object is usually the easiest task for the apraxic patient, and many who fail on verbal command and imitation will succeed with the concrete task using the real object. The presence of the object gives the patient additional visual and proprioceptive cues that facilitate performance. There are innumerable possible commands when evaluating praxis. The following are examples that will frequently elicit apraxic movements:

Buccofacial Commands

COMMANDS	ERRORS
"Show me how to—":	
1. "Blow out a match."	Difficulty giving short, controlled exhalation; saying "blow"; inhaling; difficulty maintaining appropriate mouth posture
2. "Protrude your tongue."	Inability to stick out tongue; tongue moving in mouth but tending to push against front teeth and not protruding
3. "Drink through a straw."	Inability to sustain a pucker; blowing instead of drawing through the straw; random mouthing movements

In testing buccofacial praxis, patients can often cue themselves considerably by pretending to have the object (match or straw) in their hands. This self-cuing facilitates performance and should be discouraged by gently restraining the patients' hands.

Limb Commands

COMMANDS	ERRORS
"Show me how to—":	
1. "Salute."	Hand over head; hand waving; improper position of hand

(Continued)

COMMANDS	ERRORS
2. "Use a toothbrush."	Failure to show proper grip; failure to open mouth; grossly missing the mouth; using finger to pick teeth; not allowing adequate distance for shaft of toothbrush.
3. "Flip a coin."	Movements miming tossing the coin into the air with an open hand; supinating or pronating the hand as though turning a doorknob; flexing the arm without flipping thumb against finger
4. "Hammer a nail."	Moving hand back and forth horizontally; pounding with fist
5. "Comb your hair."	Using fingers as teeth of comb; smoothing the hair; making inexact hand movements
6. "Snap your fingers."	Extension of fingers with patting movements; tapping finger on thumb; sliding finger off thumb with insufficient force
7. "Kick a ball."	Stamping foot; pushing foot along floor; moving foot laterally
8. "Crush out a cigarette."	Stamping foot; kicking foot on floor

Occasionally, apraxia is unilateral. Accordingly, commands should be alternated between left and right limbs. Do not have the patient do the same command sequentially with both hands because visual self-cuing will improve performance on the second trial.

Whole Body Commands

COMMANDS	ERRORS
"Show me how to—":	
1. "Stand like a boxer."	Awkward arm position; hands at side
2. "Swing a baseball bat."	Difficulty in placing both hands together; chopping movements
3. "Bow" [for a man] or "Curtsy" [for a woman].	Any inappropriate truncal movement

Clinical Implications

The ability to perform skilled movements on verbal command is closely associated with the language functions of the dominant hemisphere. Because adequate verbal comprehension is a prerequisite to valid praxis testing, brain area A (Fig. 9–1) must be intact. Once the command

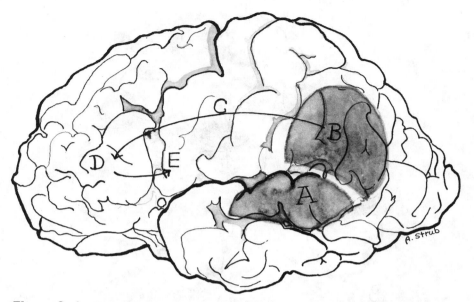

Figure 9-1. The pathways for praxis in the right hand (controlled by the left motor area).

is understood, the information spreads to the contiguous supramarginal gyrus (area B, Fig. 9-1), where the words (e.g., "flip a coin") are associated with the kinesthetic memories present in the postrolandic parietal cortex. These sensory memories of the movement are then transferred along pathway C to the premotor area (D), where memory for motor patterns is evoked. The premotor area then directs the pyramidal neurons in the motor strip (E) actually to perform the action. A lesion at any point along this pathway can cause an ideomotor apraxia. Many patients with lesions in this section of the dominant hemisphere will also be aphasic. Accordingly, praxis testing must be very carefully done to ensure that a comprehension deficit is not responsible for the impaired motor performance. In addition to these areas on the lateral surface of the left hemisphere, the supplementary motor area on the medial surface of the frontal lobe is also involved in integrating skilled limb movements. Lesions in this area in the left hemisphere can produce a bilateral limb (not buccofacial) apraxia.[44]

The foregoing paragraph outlines the pathways for praxis in the right hand (controlled by the left motor area). It has been recognized that the apraxic patient also has an apraxia with the left hand. Figure 9-2 illustrates that a command to the right motor cortex for innervation of the left hand is transferred from the left premotor area (D_1) to the right premotor area (D_2) via the anterior callosal fibers (F_1). Any interruption of this pathway will render the left hand apraxic.[24,25,45] This is often called a sympathetic dyspraxia[23] and can be readily demonstrated in the intact left hand of

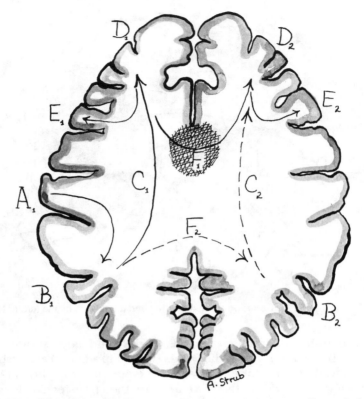

Figure 9–2. The pathways for praxis with anterior corpus callosum lesion.

patients with Broca's aphasia with right hemiplegia. Lesions of the anterior corpus callosum (F_1) will cause an isolated apraxia of the left hand; motor and praxis functions of the right hand are intact.[27] The posterior callosal pathway (F_2 to C_2), which could theoretically transmit the praxis information to the right premotor area (D_2), obviously does not.

Lesions of the right hemisphere rarely result in a significant apraxia of either hand when the patient must carry out the action to command.[14,18] Some patients with right hemisphere lesions do, however, have difficulty carrying out actions when asked to imitate the examiner.[3] In such cases the right hemisphere's stronger visual system impairs the patient's perception of the action.

This anatomic model has been verified clinically and pathologically, and firmly establishes that the hemisphere dominant for language is also dominant for learning skilled movements.[25] This dominance is obvious because most individuals have a strong hand preference for such activities as writing, throwing, and using tools. Because a lesion of the dominant hemisphere causes an apraxia in both hands, it is apparent that the dominant hemisphere exerts a continual guiding role on movements that originate from the nondominant hemisphere. Because of the close relationship between language and praxis, many aphasics have an apraxia of the buccofacial musculature. In some patients the apraxia is confined to speech movements, a condition referred to as verbal apraxia.

Not all apraxic patients demonstrate a similar degree and type of impaired performance. Some patients fail completely on command (even when comprehension of the command is adequate) yet perform perfectly on imitation. Such patients have a type of disconnection syndrome in which verbal input is literally disconnected from motor areas. Visual input, however, is relayed quickly to the motor areas, and the patient can imitate without difficulty. Most apraxic patients who fail on command, however, also have difficulty with imitation. There are some patients with ideomotor apraxia whose disorder is sufficiently severe that they fail on verbal command, on imitation, and in the use of real objects. Some patients with lesions in the left temporoparietal area seem to have considerable difficulty demonstrating the use of simple objects yet may imitate the action quite well. It has been proposed that this difficulty with real objects is an ideational apraxia rather than a severe ideomotor apraxia and is caused by a memory disorder (of object use) rather than true apraxia.[17]

Whole body commands can be performed correctly in the presence of obvious limb apraxia. They can often be accurately carried out by patients with severe auditory comprehension deficits as well. The reason for the relative sparing of performance involving whole body commands in some patients is unclear, but it may be due to the fact that these axial movements are under the control of the more widespread extrapyramidal system.[25] As a rule, however, patients with ideomotor limb apraxia also demonstrate apraxic axial movements.[37]

Ideational Apraxia

Ideational apraxia is a disturbance of complex motor planning of a higher order than is seen in ideomotor apraxia. It refers to a breakdown in performance of a task that involves a series of separate steps, such as folding a letter, placing it in an envelope, sealing it, and then placing a stamp on it. The patients can often perform each individual step of the task in isolation (e.g. folding the paper) but cannot integrate the parts accurately to complete the sequence. The patients seem to have lost the overall concept of how to go about completing the task. Some investigators define an ideational apraxia as any difficulty in manipulating real objects.[17,19] We feel that difficulty with object use in simple limb commands (e.g., inability to flip an actual coin) represents a severe ideomotor limb apraxia and not an ideational apraxia.

Evaluation

Several simple tasks are used to demonstrate an ideational apraxia:

TASKS	ERRORS
1. Folding a letter, placing it in an envelope, sealing it, addressing it, and placing a stamp on the envelope	Turning paper around without being able to fold it; folding improperly; licking the wrong side of stamp or envelope; inability to place paper in envelope
2. Placing candle in holder, taking match out of box, lighting candle, and blowing out match	Placing candle in holder wick-down; inability to place candle in holder; inability to open or close matchbox; striking match on candle; striking wrong end of match; striking candle on matchbox; blowing out candle and not match
3. Opening toothpaste, taking toothbrush from holder, and placing toothpaste on toothbrush	Removing cap from toothpaste and placing cap on toothbrush; putting toothpaste in toothbrush holder; placing toothbrush back in holder with toothpaste on it

In each of these tasks, the patient can usually perform each part of the series adequately (e.g., striking the match or brushing the teeth), but cannot coordinate the individual movements that are necessary to complete the sequence.

Clinical Implications

Ideational apraxia is a complex disability that is usually seen in patients with bilateral brain disease. Any diffuse cortical disease, especially those diseases that affect the parietal lobes, may result in an ideational apraxia. Although the patient fails on a specific task (e.g., lighting a candle), it is obvious from watching the patient's performance that his or her failure is the result of a number of cognitive deficits. Many patients have elements of ideomotor apraxia, and almost all have some degree of constructional impairment and spatial disorientation. Memory and auditory comprehension may also be diminished.

One interesting element in the performance of patients with ideational apraxia is their apparent inability to recognize the use of objects. This failure to recognize objects and their use has been called an object agnosia and may be illustrated by the patient who attempts to light a candle by striking it on the matchbox. The ability to do serial ordering is also impaired, and the complex multistep task becomes a confusing group of discrete parts with no logical, sequential relationship. The ambiguity and incongruity of the formal test situation also are confusing. The patient does not quite understand exactly what he or she is supposed to do when the doctor brings out a toothbrush and toothpaste and pushes it benignly toward the patient.

Neuropsychologically, ideational apraxia is the culmination of many significant cognitive deficits. Clinically, it results in the patient's inability to manipulate the environment effectively. The patient cannot cook a meal, make a bed, light a cigarette, put a record on the phonograph, or do any of the dozens of everyday activities that we all take for granted. Ideational apraxia is not usually a finding seen in isolation but is generally associated with widespread intellectual deterioration.

RIGHT-LEFT DISORIENTATION

Right-left orientation is traditionally defined as the ability to distinguish right from left on self and in the environment (e.g., on the examiner's body). This ability is basically a capacity for spatial orientation.[9] The application of the verbal labels "right" and "left" to the respective sides of the body is frequently used to test right-left orientation,[28] but this is a linguistic task that does not necessarily test spatial sense. Right-left disorientation may be developmental in nature or may result from either focal or diffuse brain lesions. Although this disorder is interesting and may combine with other deficits to produce Gerstmann's syndrome (discussed later in this chapter), it is of limited clinical utility when seen in isolation.

Evaluation

The following outline, which is in ascending order of difficulty, may be used to test for right-left disorientation.

TEST ITEMS
1. Identification on self
   a. Show me your right foot.
   b. Show me your left hand.
2. Crossed commands on self
   a. With your right hand touch your left shoulder.
   b. With your left hand touch your right ear.
3. Identification on examiner (with examiner facing patient)
   a. Point to my left knee.
   b. Point to my right elbow.
4. Crossed commands on examiner (with examiner facing patient)

a. With your right hand point to my left eye.
b. With your left hand point to my left foot.

Most normal persons will successfully accomplish all items without difficulty, although a significant percentage of the normal population (9% of males and over 17% of females) has demonstrable difficulty on right-left testing.[4,6]

Clinical Implications

If right-left disorientation is present, it is important to determine if the patient was ever capable of adequately performing such tasks. As previously mentioned, right-left disorientation may be developmental in nature and may also be associated with reduced general intellectual ability.

Aphasic patients may fail on right-left commands because of their primary language disorder. Anomia can cause confusion in the use of the labels "right" and "left." Deficits in auditory retention interfere with performance on complex commands.

Thus far, clinical and neuropathologic case studies have failed to demonstrate an association between right-left disorientation and any circumscribed brain lesion.[21] If an acquired disorder of right-left orientation is present, the lesion is usually located in the parietotemporal-occipital region of the dominant hemisphere.[30] In our clinical experience, right-left disorientation is infrequent in patients with lesions that are restricted to the nondominant hemisphere. This is also substantiated by Critchley's review.[9]

FINGER AGNOSIA

Finger agnosia is the inability to recognize, name, and point to individual fingers on oneself and on others.[22] This disorder may be most readily demonstrated in reference to the index, middle, and ring fingers.[8] Finger agnosia is similar to right-left orientation in that it may be developmental in nature or may result from either diffuse or focal brain disease. Its clinical utility for localization of cerebral lesions is relatively limited.

Evaluation

Evaluation of this function can be very extensive, but for practical purposes a brief screening should suffice. Patients must have adequate auditory comprehension and must know or be capable of learning the names of the fingers (thumb, index or pointing finger, middle finger, ring finger, and little finger).

TEST ITEMS
1. Nonverbal finger recognition

Directions: With the patient's eyes closed, touch one finger. Have the patient open his or her eyes and then point to the same finger on the examiner's hand.

2. Identification of named fingers on examiner's hand

Directions: The examiner's hand should be placed in various positions (e.g., palm down on the table facing the patient; hand held vertically in the air with the palm facing the patient; and hand held horizontally in the air with the palm facing the examiner). The examiner should say "Point to my middle finger," and so forth.

3. Verbal identification (naming) of fingers on self and examiner

Directions: The patient's and examiner's hands should be placed in the various positions as described earlier. The examiner points to the patient's index finger and says, "What is the name of this finger?" and so forth.

Clinical Implications

Patients with finger agnosia usually have lesions of the dominant hemisphere.[32] Left-handed patients or those with strong family histories of left-handedness may exhibit finger agnosia with lesions of either hemisphere. Parietal-occipital lesions are the most likely to cause finger agnosia.[36] As with right-left testing, aphasia will adversely affect verbally mediated performance.

With diffuse disease, finger agnosia may be seen in association with aphasia, apraxia, right-left disorientation, or general dementia. For those who desire a more comprehensive review of this topic, see Critchley[9] or Kinsbourne and Warington.[32]

GERSTMANN'S SYNDROME

Gerstmann's syndrome is a classic, albeit controversial, neurologic syndrome. It consists of four major components: finger agnosia, right-left disorientation, dysgraphia, and dyscalculia. Most patients with this disorder, however, demonstrate additional neuropsychologic deficits, principally constructional impairment or mild aphasia. The syndrome has localizing value; the demonstration of all four elements indicates damage to the dominant parietal lobe or to bilateral parietal lobes.[38,41,42] The reader who desires further information regarding this syndrome is referred to Benton,[6] Critchley,[12] and Strub and Geschwind.[42]

VISUAL AGNOSIA

Visual agnosia is a rare, acquired neurologic syndrome in which the patient is unable to recognize objects or pictures of objects presented visually. Visual acuity is adequate, mentation clear, and aphasia absent.[43]

Two major categories of visual agnosia have been described in the literature. In the first type, actual visual perception of the object is distorted to the point that recognition is impossible. Such patients cannot name or tell the use of an object when it is shown to them but can readily name and demonstrate the use of the object when it is placed in their hands. Kinesthetic cues provide sufficient information for recognition. To evaluate for the presence of visual agnosia, ask the patient to identify verbally common objects presented visually. If the patient fails to recognize the object, allow manipulation of the object. If the patient then readily identifies the object, the defect is in the visual system. It has been postulated that such patients have damage to the visual association cortex bilaterally (areas 18 and 19). This type of visual agnosia (apperceptive visual agnosia) has been reported in a patient with anoxic encephalopathy secondary to carbon dioxide poisoning.[5]

The second variety of visual agnosia is called associative visual agnosia. Patients with this type of agnosia have adequate visual perception but their visual cortex is disconnected from the language area or visual memory stores. Accordingly, they can recognize the object and demonstrate its use, but they cannot name it. When unable to name an object, such patients are also unable to describe its use.[40] The evaluation for this disorder is similar to that for the first type of visual agnosia, except that adequate visual perception must be demonstrated. This can be done with a simple visual matching task. Lesions that cause an associative visual agnosia may be bilateral, involving the inferior temporal occipital junction and subjacent white matter,[2] or may be an infarct that destroys the left occipital lobe and the posterior corpus callosum.[33] This is the same lesion that causes alexia without agraphia, and, in fact, most patients with associative visual agnosia are also alexic. For further reading, refer to Critchley,[10] Bender and Feldman,[4] Lhermitte and Beauvois,[33] Albert, Reches, and Silverberg,[1] and Alexander and Albert.[2]

Two additional types of visual agnosia deserve mention but will not be fully discussed. Prosopagnosia is an unusual agnosia in which patients are unable to recognize familiar faces. In such cases, the agnosia is so profound that even members of the patient's immediate family are not recognized. The patient will recognize the person, however, on hearing his or her voice. The mechanism that results in prosopagnosia is probably a combination of a disturbance of fine visual discrimination and a failure of memory for the discrete category of human faces. The lesions that are responsible for this disorder are usually in the occipitotemporal areas bilaterally. One of the lesions is usually in the right inferior temporo-occipital region.[34] For further references, see DeRenzi and Spinnler,[20] Benton and Van Allen,[7] Meadows,[34] or Damasio, Damasio, and Van Hoesen.[13]

Color agnosia is an inability to recognize colors secondary to an acquired cortical lesion. Two types of color agnosia have been described.

There is a specific color-naming disturbance that results from a discon-nection of visual input from the language area. This anomia is associated with the syndrome of alexia with agraphia.[26] In this form, there is no dam-age to the primary language area and no other evidence of aphasia.

The second and more common disturbance of color recognition is actually a defect in color perception caused by bilateral inferior temporo-occipital lesions. These are the same lesions that cause prosopagnosia, and most patients with this type of color agnosia have concomitant pro-sopagnosia.[35] For further reading on this topic, refer to Critchley[11] and DeRenzi and associates.[16]

ASTEREOGNOSIS

Stereognosis is the ability to discriminate the size and shape of objects and to identify them by touch alone. This is usually tested during the routine neurologic examination by asking the patient to identify several common objects placed in his or her hand (e.g., coin, key, paperclip, and so forth). The patient is tested with the eyes closed and is given one object at a time. The patient is allowed to manipulate the object freely. Each hand is tested individually.[9,29]

The task demands that the patient be able to integrate spatial features and weight and texture in order to identify the object. If a patient has a defect in primary sensation in the hand, failure to identify the object cannot be attributed to astereognosis.

Astereognosis, or a failure of tactile recognition, is usually indicative of a lesion in the anterior portion of the parietal lobe opposite the aster-eognostic hand.[39] the lesion involves the postcentral gyrus. Cases have been reported in which a unilateral lesion, either right or left, produced a bilateral defect.[9] A rare form of left-hand unilateral astereognosis has been reported in patients with a lesion in the anterior corpus callosum.[27]

GEOGRAPHIC DISORIENTATION

Geographic orientation is a complex ability that includes the patient's capacity to find his or her way in familiar environments, to localize places on maps or floor plans, and to find his or her way in new environments. A significant geographic disorientation will interfere with the patient's abil-ity to live a normal life. Such patients are unable to travel alone outside of their home and may even become disoriented within their own houses.

Evaluation

History Obtained from Family

In evaluating geographic orientation, it is important to obtain historic information regarding the patient's ability to operate in familiar and unfamiliar environments outside of the formal testing situation. Such information is best obtained from family members rather than from the patient.

1. Does the patient become lost at work, in the neighborhood, or at home?
2. Has the patient become lost traveling to a less-frequented location (e.g., the inability to locate a restaurant not visited in a year)?
3. Does the patient have great difficulty orienting to new environments?

Localizing Places on a Map

Map localization is an abstract task that can quickly detect disturbances in geographic orientation. It is also useful when adequate historic information is unobtainable, and it may bring out subtle defects in unilateral attention.[8]

Directions: Have the patient draw a map of the United States. If he or she is unable to produce a recognizable representation, the doctor should draw one or provide a suitable outline. Ask the patient to localize the following cities on the map outline:

1. Denver
2. New York
3. San Francisco
4. New Orleans
5. Chicago

Scoring: In reviewing the patient's performance, the following factors should be considered: (1) Are coastal cities located on the coast? (2) Are the cities in the appropriate states? (3) Are all cities in one half of the map (either east or west)? (4) Are attempts made to localize all cities?

Ability to Orient Self in Hospital Environment

Information concerning the patient's ability to orient himself or herself in the hospital may be obtained from nurses' reports and by observing the patient's capacity to find his or her bed, ward, and bathroom. For example, we saw a patient with communicating hydrocephalus and mild dementia who, on concluding a fifth office revisit, walked confidently into the closet.

Clinical Implications

Geographic disorientation has been clinically associated with parietal lobe disease,[9] although few good clinicoanatomic studies have been reported. Of the studies available, there is some suggestion that right hemisphere lesions most frequently cause geographic difficulty.[31] Other studies, however, have failed to support this finding of lateralization and report an approximately equal incidence of geographic disorientation in patients with right and left hemisphere lesions.[8]

A consistent finding of clinical utility is that patients with unilateral lesions tend to localize cities on the map toward the side of their lesion (e.g., patients with left parietal lesions tend to place cities toward the west coast on the map outline). This appears to be a result of neglect of the contralateral visual field.[8] A more generalized geographic disorientation is a frequent finding in patients with diffuse cortical disease and may be an early sign of dementing illness.

Geographic orientation is probably not a unitary cortical function but a combination of more basic cognitive processes including visual memory, right-left orientation, visual perception, and spatial neglect. Performance on formal tests of geographic orientation, such as locating cities on a map outline, is closely associated with both general intelligence and social exposure (education). General lack of geographic knowledge is the most common cause of failure on this test and we were surprised to find that our normal subjects (on an average) only correctly located half of the five cities requested.

One must not minimize the devastating effects that clinically significant geographic disorientation has on the patient's ability to function effectively in his or her environment. Such patients are typically unable to work, easily become lost in unfamiliar places, and eventually have difficulty with orientation in even familiar settings such as the neighborhood and home.

SUMMARY

The cortical functions of apraxia, visual and finger agnosia, astereognosis, geographic disorientation, and right-left disorientation are interesting and may be clinically relevant in localizing brain lesions.

REFERENCES

1. Albert, ML, Reches, A, and Silverberg, R: Associative visual agnosia without alexia. Neurology 25:322, 1975.
2. Alexander, MF and Albert, ML: The anatomical basis of visual agnosia. In Kertesz, A (ed): Localization in Neuropsychology. Academic Press, New York, 1983, pp 393–415.
3. Barbieri, C and DeRenzi, E: The executive and ideational components of apraxia. Cortex 24:535, 1988.
4. Bender, M and Feldman, M: The so-called "visual agnosias." Brain 95:173, 1972.
5. Benson, DF and Greenberg, J: Visual form agnosia. Arch Neurol 20:82, 1969.
6. Benton, A: The fiction of the Gerstmann syndrome. J Neurol Neurosurg Psychiatry 24:176, 1961.
7. Benton, A and Van Allen, M: Prosopagnosia and facial discrimination. J Neurol Sci 15:167, 1972.
8. Benton, A, Levin, H, and Van Allen, M: Geographic orientation in patients with unilateral cerebral disease. Neuropsychologia 12:183, 1974.

9. Critchley, M: The Parietal Lobes. Hafner, New York, 1966.
10. Critchley, M: The problem of visual agnosia. J Neurol Sci 1:274, 1964.
11. Critchley, M: Acquired anomalies of colour perception of central origin. Brain 88:711, 1965.
12. Critchley, M: The enigma of Gerstmann's syndrome. Brain 89:183, 1966.
13. Damasio, AR, Damasio, H, and Van Hoesen, GW: Prosopagnosia: Anatomic basis and behavioral mechanisms. Neurology 32:331, 1982.
14. DeAjuriaguerra, J, Hécaen, H, and Angelerques, R: Les apraxies: Varietes cliniques et lateralisation lesionnelle. Rev Neurol 102:566, 1960.
15. Denny-Brown, D: The nature of apraxia. J Nerv Ment Dis 126:9, 1958.
16. DeRenzi, E, et al: Impairment in associating colour to form, concomitant with aphasia. Brain 95:293, 1972.
17. DeRenzi, E and Lucchelli, F: Ideational apraxia. Brain 111:1173, 1988.
18. DeRenzi, E, Motti, F, and Nichelli, P: Imitating gestures: A quantitative approach to ideo-motor apraxia. Arch Neurol 37:6 1980.
19. DeRenzi, E, Pieczuro, A, and Vignolo, L: Ideational apraxia: A quantitative study. Neuropsychologia 6:41, 1968.
20. DeRenzi, E and Spinnler, H: Facial recognition in brain damaged patients. Neurology 16:145, 1966.
21. Frederiks, J: Disorders of the body schema. In Vinken, P and Bruyn, G (eds): Handbook of Clinical Neurology, Vol 4, Disorders of Speech, Perception and Symbolic Behavior. American Elsevier, New York, 1969, pp 207–240.
22. Gerstmann, J: Some notes on the Gerstmann-syndrome. Neurology 7:866, 1957.
23. Geschwind, N: Sympathetic dyspraxia. Trans Am Neurol Assoc 88:219, 1963.
24. Geschwind, N: Disconnection syndromes in animals and man, Part II. Brain 88:585, 1965.
25. Geschwind, N: The apraxias: Neural mechanisms of disorders of learned movement. Am Sci 63:188, 1975.
26. Geschwind, N and Fusillo, M: Color-naming defects in association with alexia. Arch Neurol 15:137, 1966.
27. Geschwind, N and Kaplan, E: A human cerebral deconnection syndrome. Neurology 12:675, 1962.
28. Goodglass, H and Kaplan, E: The Assessment of Aphasia and Related Disorders, ed 2. Lea & Febiger, Philadelphia, 1983.
29. Hécaen, H and Albert, ML: Human Neuropsychology. John Wiley & Sons, 1978, pp 297–303.
30. Hécaen, H and DeAjuriaguerra, J: Meconnaissances et Hallucinations Corporelles. Masson et Cie, Paris, 1952.
31. Hécaen, H and Angelerques, R: La Cecite Psychique. Masson et Cie, Paris, 1963.
32. Knisbourne, M and Warrington, E: A study of finger agnosia. Brain 85:47, 1962.
33. Lhermitte, F and Beauvois, M: A visual-speech disconnection syndrome. Brain 96:695, 1973.
34. Meadows, J: The anatomical basis of prosopagnosia. J Neurol Neurosurg Psychiatry 37:489, 1974.
35. Meadows, J: Disturbed perception of colours associated with localized cerebral lesions. Brain 97:615, 1974.
36. Nielsen, J: Gerstmann syndrome: Finger agnosia, agraphia, confusion of right and left, and acalculia. Arch Neurol Psychiatry 39:536, 1983.
37. Poeck, K, Lehmkuhl, G, and Willmes, K: Axial movements in ideomotor apraxia. J Neurol Neurosurg Psychiatry 45:1125, 1982.
38. Roeltgen, DP, Sevush, S, and Heilman, KM: Pure Gerstmann's syndrome from a focal lesion. Arch Neurol 40:46, 1983.
39. Roland, PE: Focal increase of cerebral blood flow during stereognostic testing in man. Arch Neurol 33:543, 1976.

40. Rubens, A and Benson, DF: Associative visual agnosia. Arch Neurol 24:305, 1971.
41. Strub, RL and Geschwind, N: Gerstmann syndrome without aphasia. Cortex 10:378, 1974.
42. Strub, RL and Geschwind, N: Localization in Gerstmann syndrome. In Kertesz, A (ed): Localization in Neuropsychology. Academic Press, New York, 1983, pp 295–321.
43. Warrington, EK: Agnosia: The impairment of object recognition. In Frederiks, JAM (ed): Handbook of Clinical Neurology, Vol 1(45), Clinical Neuropsychology. Elsevier Science, Amsterdam, 1985, pp 333–349.
44. Watson, RT, et al: Apraxia and the supplementary area. Arch Neurol 43:787, 1986.
45. Watson, RT and Heilman, KM: Callosal apraxia. Brain 106:391, 1983.
46. Wolf, SM: Difficulties in right-left discrimination in a normal population. Arch Neurol 29:128, 1973.

Chapter 10

Summary of Examination

Throughout this book, we have emphasized the importance of performing a systematic and complete mental status examination. Although it is not always necessary to evaluate exhaustively every aspect of mental functioning, certain critical functions should be assessed in every patient. These include level of consciousness, physical appearance and emotional status, attention, expressive and receptive language, memory, constructional ability, and abstract reasoning. Items that are adequate for evaluating these areas are shown with an asterisk in the composite mental status examination shown in Appendix 2.

The experienced clinician is able to tailor the mental status examination to the individual patient's clinical problem, and with practice, an adequate screening examination can be completed in 15 to 30 minutes. In patients for whom the history of behavioral complaints is vague, or when emotional features predominate, a more extensive examination may be required.

The systematic mental status examination usually allows the clinician to differentiate accurately patients with organic brain disease from both normal persons and those with functional disorders. In many cases, it is also possible to specify the type, locus, and degree of disease. For example, knowledge of specific patterns of aphasia often permits the examiner to localize a lesion within the dominant hemisphere. In other cases, the pattern of performance is suggestive of a specific disease entity (e.g., Alzheimer's disease).

In the clinical implications sections of each chapter in this book, we have attempted to describe many neurobehavioral syndromes as they relate to specific areas of cognitive deficit. Examples of these are the acute confusional states (Chapter 2), aphasias and related language disorders (Chapter 5), amnesias (Chapter 6), and the frontal lobe syndrome (Chapter 2). These clinical implications sections are not intended to be a comprehensive review of neurobehavior or an intensive discussion of any one syndrome. They are, rather, illustrations of the bridge between the data and the diagnosis. See Strub and Black[4] for a complete discussion of these topics.

In general, the more clinical data the examiner obtains regarding the patient's level of functioning in a variety of areas, the more accurate the final diagnosis will be. An examination that includes all of the items discussed in this book and outlined in Appendix 2 can usually be completed in an hour or less. Although all of the data are valuable, the busy physician may not always be able to spend this much time on all routine consultations. In most clinical settings, the physician is initially interested in making a tentative diagnosis and planning an appropriate diagnostic evaluation; therefore, he or she will tailor the examination to fit the clinical situation. Following are discussions of several specific clinical neurobehavioral syndromes. Because of the magnitude of the problem of dementia, a disproportionate amount of space is devoted to the use of the mental status examination in diagnosing that condition.

ALZHEIMER'S DISEASE

One of the most common organic brain disorders is dementia.[2] Alzheimer's disease (senile dementia Alzheimer type [SDAT]) is the most prevalent and well-known cause.[2,3,5] Even though effective treatment is not yet available, it is important to recognize the early features of this syndrome because early diagnosis can prevent serious social and vocational embarrassment to both patient and family. The early features of this disease, which can readily be demonstrated on a systematic mental status examination, are apathy, vague subjective complaints, memory difficulties, constructional impairment, dyscalculia (calculation problems), and problems with abstract reasoning. As the disease progresses, anomia, apraxia, agnosia, geographic disorientation, and significant deficits in judgment typically appear, and those defects seen in the early stages worsen. In the deteriorated stage, all deficits are accentuated, behavior is regressed, language, memory, and thought processes are severely disturbed, and the patient requires total care. The diagnosis of Alzheimer's disease in the advanced stages is usually made without difficulty, but it is surprising how often mild but significant dementia goes unrecognized by family and physician alike.

The mental status examination for a patient with suspected dementia (Table 10–1) can be shortened, but it should include the following essential components:

1. *Level of consciousness:* Patients with simple atrophic dementia (Alzheimer's and senile Alzheimer's disease) are fully alert unless they have a secondary decrease in the level of consciousness from medication, medical illness, or a focal brain lesion with increased intracranial pressure.
2. *Behavior observations:* These are important, but as they are made throughout the history and examination, they will rarely prolong the examination time.
3. *Language:* Spontaneous speech and comprehension can be roughly assessed during history taking, but repetition and naming should

Table 10–1 MENTAL STATUS EXAMINATION FOR DEMENTIA

PATIENT INFORMATION

NAME: DATE:

HOSPITAL OR FILE NUMBER:

AGE: SEX: DIAGNOSIS:

1. VERBAL FLUENCY

    Animals per 60 seconds   Total animals: _____

2. COMPREHENSION   Check if correct:

    a. Point to the ceiling.   _____

    b. Point to your nose and window.   _____

    c. Point to your foot, door, and ceiling.   _____

    d. Point to window, leg, door, and thumb.   _____

3. NAMING AND WORD FINDING

    Parts of objects: Watch stem (winder)   _____

                             Coat lapel   _____

                             Watch crystal   _____

                             Sole of shoe   _____

                             Buckle of belt   _____

4. ORIENTATION

    a. Date   _____

    b. Month   _____

    c. Year   _____

    d. Day of week   _____

5. NEW LEARNING ABILITY

    Four unrelated words: 5 min   10 min

    a. Brown (Fun)   _____   _____

    b. Honesty (Loyalty)   _____   _____

    c. Tulip (Carrot)   _____   _____

    d. Eyedropper (Ankle)   _____   _____

(Continued)

Table 10–1 *(continued)*

6. VERBAL STORY FOR IMMEDIATE RECALL

   It was July/ and the Rogers/ had packed up/ their four children/ in the station wagon/ and were off/ on vacation.

   They were taking/ their yearly trip/ to the beach/ at Gulf Shores.

   This year/ they were making/ a special/ one-day stop/ at The Aquarium/ in New Orleans.

   After a long day's drive/ they arrived/ at the motel/ only to discover/ that in their excitement/ they had left/ the twins/ and their suitcases/ in the front yard.

   Number of correct memories: _____

7. VISUAL MEMORY (HIDDEN OBJECTS)

Object	Found
a. Coin	_____
b. Pen	_____
c. Comb	_____
d. Key	_____
e. Fork	_____

8. PAIRED ASSOCIATE LEARNING

1	2
a. Weather-Bag	a. House-Income
b. High-Low	b. Weather-Bag
c. House-Income	c. Book-Page
d. Book-Page	d. High-Low

1	2
a. House _____	a. High _____
b. High _____	a. House _____
c. Weather _____	c. Book _____
d. Book _____	d. Weather _____

9. CONSTRUCTIONAL ABILITY

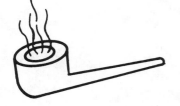

   Score _____

(Continued)

Table 10–1 *(continued)*

Daisy in flower pot   Score _____

House in perspective   Score _____

10. WRITTEN COMPLEX
    CALCULATIONS

    a.   Addition
$$\begin{array}{r} 108 \\ +\ 79 \\ \hline \end{array}$$

    b.   Subtraction
$$\begin{array}{r} 605 \\ -\ 86 \\ \hline \end{array}$$

    c.   Multiplication
$$\begin{array}{r} 108 \\ \times\ 36 \\ \hline \end{array}$$

    d.   Division $43\overline{)559}$ Number correct _____

(Continued)

Table 10–1 *(continued)*

11. PROVERB INTERPRETATION

    a. Don't cry over spilled milk.   Score

    _____   _____

    b. Rome wasn't built in a day.

    _____   _____

    c. A drowning man will clutch at a straw.

    _____   _____

    d. A golden hammer breaks an iron door.

    _____   _____

    e. The hot coal burns, the cold one blackens.

    _____   _____

12. SIMILARITIES

    a. Turnip .... Cauliflower   _____
    b. Car .... Airplane   _____
    c. Desk .... Bookcase   _____
    d. Poem .... Novel   _____
    e. Horse .... Apple   _____

be specifically tested. Although naming and word-finding errors are often present in patients with dementia, repetition is usually intact unless the disease is advanced or there is an associated left hemisphere lesion with aphasia.

    4. *Memory:* This is a critical term. Orientation should be tested first. If the patient fails, particularly if it is a significant failure, this strongly suggests a new-learning or recent-memory deficit. Next, tell the patient the correct date and location and ask him or her to remember it. Then ask about recent news items for a few minutes, and then ask the orientation questions again. If there is a second failure, in our experience the patient has a significant memory problem and additional testing will only support this initial impression and will not provide additional substantive data. If the patient is

oriented or quickly learns his or her orientation, carry out the full memory section of the examination.

5. *Drawings:* These take only a few minutes to perform and are an invaluable aid in diagnosing brain disease, especially dementia.
6. *Abstract functions:*
   Calculations: These are very useful when evaluating demented patients; several examples should be included.
   Proverbs and similarities: These are also useful, and several of each should be asked. The demented patient tends to answer in a very concrete manner.

After many years of use and statistic analysis of several hundred cases of Alzheimer's disease, the shortened form of the mental status examination shown on Table 10–1 was developed. The items were selected on the basis of sensitivity in diagnosing dementia. These items are not specific to Alzheimer's disease but are highly likely to be abnormal in that population (i.e., highly sensitive). The total score for this test is 100 points (Table 10–2). As there is the potential for false-positive results (i.e., diagnosing dementia in nondemented individuals) in the elderly, a total score in the 50 to 60 range in an 85-year-old must be cautiously interpreted (Table 10–3).

ACUTE CONFUSIONAL STATE

A history of a rapid decrease in mental status (hours to a few days) does not usually suggest a primary dementia but more likely a delirium (acute confusional state). As discussed in Chapter 2, this condition is usually easily recognized by its typical behavioral features and represents a specific diagnostic entity. Extensive mental status testing will be abnormal but rarely adds additional useful diagnostic information.

DOMINANT HEMISPHERE LESIONS

Patients with lesions of the dominant hemisphere will frequently show abnormalities of language functions. In the right-handed patient, evidence of aphasia, alexia, or agraphia almost always indicates left hemisphere disease. Gerstmann's syndrome, constructional impairment, verbal memory difficulties, ideomotor apraxia, dyscalculia, and impairment of verbal reasoning are all findings that can be seen with left hemisphere lesions. Denial and neglect are not commonly seen in these patients. Even left-handed patients will frequently show the aforementioned findings with left hemisphere disease, although there is a higher frequency of bilateral representation of these functions in these patients.

Table 10–2. MENTAL STATUS SCORESHEET

PATIENT:		Score
Verbal fluency—animal names (1 point/2 animals)	Maximum: 10 points	_____
Verbal comprehension (pointing)	4 points	_____
Naming—parts of objects	5 points	_____

Memory

Orientation: Date 2 points Day 2 points Month 1 point Year 1 point	6 points	_____
Unrelated words (2 points each) 5 min _____ 10 min _____	16 points	_____
Story (1 point = 1 remembered item [13 maximum])	13 points	_____
Hidden objects (1 point each)	5 points	_____
Paired associate learning	8 points	_____

Drawings Pipe, daisy, house	9 points	_____
Calculations (written)	4 points	_____
Proverbs	10 points	_____
Similarities	10 points	_____
	Maximum: 100 points	_____

Table 10–3. TOTAL SCORES ON MENTAL STATUS EXAMINATION FOR DEMENTIA*

NORMAL INDIVIDUALS (BY AGE GROUP)					PATIENTS WITH ALZHEIMER'S DISEASE (BY STAGE)		
40–49	50–59	60–69	70–79	80–89	I	II	III
80.9 (9.7)	82.3 (8.6)	75.5 (10.5)	66.9 (9.1)	67.9 (11.0)	57.2 (9.1)	37.0 (7.8)	13.4 (8.1)

*Mean ± Standard deviation.

NONDOMINANT HEMISPHERE LESIONS

Although most patients with lesions of the nondominant hemisphere do not show evidence of language disorders, they do have a more dramatic constructional impairment than do patients with dominant hemisphere lesions. In such patients, denial and neglect are more common and severe in degree, malalignment is seen in writing and calculations, and deficits are present in nonverbal memory.

RECORDING, SUMMARIZING, AND INTERPRETING DATA

As with any medical examination, it is very important to record both what was specifically tested and the patient's responses to each item. To aid in recording these data, a form similar to the composite in Appendix 2 should be used. At the completion of the examination, the clinician should synthesize the data and then summarize and emphasize the key areas of impairment. This summary allows an identification of deficit patterns and the efficient communication of essential findings.

The clinician must summarize and organize the data in such a way that he or she can arrive at the following four clinical implications:

1. *Describe the major areas of impairment:* Indicate those areas of mental status functioning that are deficient compared with the level expected in the patient, based on his or her education and premorbid function. This implies a deficit in a general area of functioning (e.g., verbal memory, abstraction, or construction ability) rather than an abnormality on an individual test (e.g., paired associate learning). This is the initial step in organizing the data so that they can be interpreted neurobehaviorally.

2. *Make a tentative neurobehavioral diagnosis:* Having indicated the major areas of impairment, the clinician can now analyze the pattern of deficits and make a specific neurobehavioral diagnosis: delirium, dementia, organic amnesic state, aphasia, nondominant hemisphere syndrome, and so forth. The interpretation of the mental status findings is difficult and, as in all fields of medicine, requires clinical experience with patients who have organic brain syndromes (neurobehavioral disorders), as well as additional reading in this area.

3. *Arrive at a tentative localization of the lesion:* This step is of both practical and academic importance. In a practical sense, findings that suggest a single focal lesion (e.g., fluent aphasia without other deficits, suggesting a left temporal or temporoparietal lesion) require a far different neurodiagnostic evaluation than does the identification of an acute confusional state. Academically it is of great

interest to attempt to correlate clinical findings with what is known about brain function.

4. *Make a tentative clinical diagnosis:* This is the final step in the diagnostic process. It requires the clinician to correlate historic and examination data with medical knowledge to make a specific medical diagnosis. For example, a patient with a slowly developing cognitive deterioration, whose mental status examination shows multiple areas of impairment suggesting bilateral brain disease (dementia), yet who has normal results on a standard neurologic examination, most likely has Alzheimer's disease. Similarly, an elderly patient with the acute onset of aphasia with fluent paraphasic speech with impaired comprehension (Wernicke's aphasia) probably has had an occlusion of a posterior branch of the left middle cerebral artery.

This entire summary process requires careful thought and considerable clinical knowledge. When the examiner becomes proficient with the examination and familiar with the organic syndromes, this complex process of data analysis and diagnosis becomes easier.

The final steps in any patient evaluation include communicating test findings to the patient, the patient's family, and the referring physician; referring the patient for further evaluation when necessary; and arranging for appropriate subsequent patient management.

CONCLUSION

As stated in our introduction, we have intended to help the clinician to understand many of the cognitive functions that can be easily tested at the bedside. We have tried to give enough information concerning these functions and their disturbance in brain disease to allow the examiner to test the patient and to delineate the deficits. Understanding these deficits and how to test for them, and recognizing the common pattern in disease, frequently will allow the examiner to make a specific diagnosis.

After reading this book, the neurologist, psychiatrist, psychologist, or general physician should be able to conduct a comprehensive examination of the patient with brain disease and use the data for diagnosis. Although this mental status examination is qualitative in nature, it can be quantitative if the examiner so desires. Some screening tests (the "mini-mental state"[1] being the most widely used) will give the examiner a single score, which is used to identify the presence and degree of organic disease. This quantitative method, in contrast to the comprehensive qualitative examination, can provide only a gross estimate of the patient's global cognitive functioning and is restricted in its contents, scope, and sensitivity. We do not believe that professionals in the field of behavior (i.e., neurologists, psychiatrists, psychologists, and so forth) should rely solely on this type of gross screening test.

REFERENCES

1. Folstein, MF, Folstein, SE, and McHugh, PR: "Mini-Mental State": A practical method for grading the cognitive state of patients for the clinician. J Psychiatr Res 12:189, 1975.
2. Katzman, R: The prevalence and malignancy of Alzheimer's disease. Arch Neurol 33:217, 1976.
3. Katzman, R and Karasu, T: Differential diagnosis of dementia. In Fields, W (ed): Neurological and Sensory Disorders in the Elderly. Stratton Intercontinental Medical Book, New York, 1975, pp 103–134.
4. Strub, RL and Black FW: Neurobehavioral Disorders: A Clinical Approach. FA Davis, Philadelphia, 1988.
5. Whitehouse, PJ (ed): Dementia. FA Davis, Philadelphia, 1992.

Chapter 11

Further Evaluations

After completion of the routine mental status examination, in a number of situations additional evaluation is warranted. This section briefly discusses the contributions of the neuropsychologist, speech pathologist, psychiatrist, and social worker to the total evaluation of the patient with organic brain disease. Despite the important contributions of such specialists, it is beyond the scope of this book to offer more than an introduction and suggested readings.

NEUROPSYCHOLOGY

The clinical neuropsychologist is trained at the doctoral level, with a 1-year clinical internship or a postdoctoral fellowship, or both, during which formal training is given in the use and interpretation of standard psychologic tests and specialized neuropsychologic procedures to evaluate patients with organic brain disease. The International Neuropsychological Society/American Psychological Association Neuropsychology Task Force on Education now recommends a 2-year fellowship training program following the internship year. This training usually includes neuroanatomy, physiology, and basic clinical neurology, in addition to topics of a more traditional psychologic nature. The clinical neuropsychologist is primarily concerned with the identification, description, and quantification of changes in behavior (cognitive, motor, and emotional) that are associated with brain dysfunction. Because of the specialized training, the clinical neuropsychologist's primary area of interest and expertise is the relationships between human behavior (whether specific to a response on a formal test or in general) and brain function and dysfunction. Accordingly, the neuropsychologist can aid in a variety of important clinical problems, including differential diagnosis, lateralization and localization of lesions, establishment of baselines of behavior and cognitive performance from which improvement or deterioration can be gauged, determination of competence in the aged or demented, and development of remedial methods for the rehabilitation of the individual brain-damaged patient.[9,10,23,29,32,36]

The neuropsychologic evaluation is a comprehensive, objective assessment of a wide range of cognitive, adaptive, and emotional behaviors that reflect the adequacy (or inadequacy) of higher brain functions. In essence, the neuropsychologic evaluation is a greatly expanded and objectified mental status examination. Whereas the mental status examination is designed to screen a variety of critical areas briefly, the neuropsychologic evaluation assesses a wider range of performance in more depth over a longer period (3 to 8 hours). It differs from the mental status examination in that it generally uses tests and evaluation procedures that have been standardized with samples of either normal people or brain-damaged patients. Because of this use of standardized measures, comparisons can be made between the individual patient's performance and that of standardized normative groups. Additionally, the varying adequacy of the same patients' performance can be compared across a variety of cognitive areas. The objective and highly quantified nature of most neuropsychologic tests aids in the detection of subtle changes in performance over time (e.g., the slowly deteriorating dementia or the improvement in specific functions after neurosurgery). Because of the wide range of behaviors assessed and the depth to which they are evaluated, the neuropsychologic evaluation may detect subtle deficits not apparent on the mental status examination.

The neuropsychologic evaluation has a number of advantages not shared by many standard neurodiagnostic techniques. It is noninvasive, with no risk of mortality or morbidity, and the evaluation provides important descriptive and prognostic information that other techniques cannot. This is especially true with regard to a description of the effects of neurologic disease on the patient as a person and its probable impact on academic, social, and vocational adjustment. The functional effects of brain disease or injury can be documented only with neuropsychologic assessment.

The physician without ready access to a trained neuropsychologist may consult a clinical psychologist who has had supervised experience in evaluating patients with brain damage. A review of the information contained in this section and in the appendix of neuropsychologic tests should greatly aid in interpreting the final reports received from such a psychologist.

A common feature of the psychologic reports that are provided by persons other than neuropsychologists, which may be difficult to interpret without some knowledge of their meaning, is the frequent reporting of so-called organic signs. Such signs typically include:

1. Verbal-performance discrepancies (e.g., appreciable differences between the verbal IQ and performance IQ on the Wechsler series of intelligence tests). Differences exceeding 25 points are statistically significant,[8] although those of 15 points are of some clinical utility in suggesting neurologic dysfunction.[4,5] Reported verbal and performance discrepancies must be cautiously interpreted in light of the overall psychologic test profile, any primary sensory or motor deficit (e.g., a visual impairment or cerebral palsy), the patient's

educational and language background, and the relatively high base rate of significant discrepancies in the general population.[24]

2. A scattering of performance levels on the various subtests of the Wechsler tests or among any scores obtained from the full psychologic test battery (e.g., a subtest score of 12 on the Wechsler's Adult Intelligence Scale [WAIS] Vocabulary Subtest and 6 on the Similarities Subtest). Such differential performance does indicate discrepant intellectual functioning that must be explained. The physician should recognize, however, that a number of factors (social, psychologic, and educational) other than brain damage may result in such subtest scatter. Accordingly, this sign should not be interpreted in isolation as indicating brain damage.

3. An indication of visuomotor dysfunction as detected by any measure of constructional ability, including the nonverbal WAIS subtests, the Bender's gestalt test, drawings to command, and so forth. The best predictors of brain damage on such tests are specific errors of rotation and perseveration. Errors related to the integration of parts or the distortion of elements of the gestalt tend to be maturational rather than pathologic. A wide variety of social, maturational, motor, and sensory factors, as well as brain damage, may impinge on constructional ability; thus, information regarding performance in this area must be evaluated within the context of the total psychologic evaluation and the patient's history. Constructional ability and its impairment are covered in depth in Chapter 7.

In sum, the information provided by the clinical psychologist may be valuable to the physician in describing the abilities and disabilities of the patient and in helping to document the effects of brain damage. The referring physician must, however, use the services of a well-trained and experienced psychologist, must understand something of the nature of the commonly employed psychologic tests, and must be able to interpret both the utility and the many limitations of the so-called brain damage indicators or organic signs. Because of the rapid expansion of clinical neuropsychology since the previous edition of this book, access to formally trained neuropsychologists has significantly increased, especially in urban centers and medium-sized cities.

Referral

Appropriate referrals for neuropsychologic evaluation include patients in whom brain damage is suspected, but not unequivocally verified, as well as those for whom the physician requires further information regarding diagnosis, description of the effects of a well-verified lesion on behavior, or prognosis and management. As with any consultation, the referring physician should state as clearly as possible what question(s) need answering (e.g., "Is this patient demented or depressed?" or "Will this head injury interfere with the patient's ability to do his or her job?").

Cognitive and behavioral disturbances may occur in the absence of any clear-cut physical signs of cerebral disease on a standard clinical neurologic examination; this is particularly true in cases of early dementia. Patients with dementia typically present initially with vague behavioral complaints such as mental dullness, concentration problems, increasing apathy, loss of interest in job or family, chronic fatigue, depression, and subjective memory problems. The neuropsychologic evaluation of such patients can often contribute along with other neurodiagnostic procedures, to an early diagnosis. The common diagnostic problem of differentiating between dementia and depression is frequently solved by the data obtained from the neuropsychologic battery. In other cases, the neuropsychologic evaluation may provide initial data suggestive of brain dysfunction and thus may serve as a basis for ordering more extensive and specific neurodiagnostic procedures.

The evaluation can also determine the relative impact of the organic and functional components in a patient with mixed neurologic and psychiatric complaints.

Any patient with a documented brain lesion in whom rehabilitation is planned should receive a complete neuropsychologic assessment as part of the total evaluation. The comprehensive nature of the evaluation will provide valuable information regarding the effect of the lesion on cognitive functioning, emotional status, behavior, and social adjustment. Objective data document both specific areas of impairment and residual abilities. This outline of strengths and weaknesses is essential in describing the effects of specific neurologic disorders on the patient's functioning, and provides information that is critical for vocational and social rehabilitation.

Periodic reevaluation can provide reliable, objective information regarding the speed and degree of recovery after brain injury or after neurosurgical procedures and specific drug treatment regimens. Similarly, repeat evaluations can be used to assess deterioration in cases of progressive disease or to rule out such progression in equivocal cases. Preneurosurgical and postneurosurgical testing will help to quantify the effects of surgery on the cognitive, behavioral, vocational, and social functioning of the patient. In a similar sense, the effects of any medical treatment (e.g., the use of levodopa in parkinsonism or anticonvulsants in epilepsy) can be well documented by pretreatment and posttreatment neuropsychologic evaluation. These changes over time are difficult to assess without an adequate baseline of objective data.

In any case of trauma or suspected brain damage involving litigation or compensation, the objective data obtained from neuropsychologic evaluation are obviously of great value in documenting and describing the presence, absence, or degree of disability. There is considerable legal precedent for the admission of testimony of psychologists as expert witnesses in such cases.[7] Forensic neuropsychology is a rapidly emerging subspecialty that can prove very helpful to the clinician and attorney dealing with cases of traumatically acquired brain damage.[7,25,37]

Neuropsychologic Evaluation

The following is a summary of the clinical services that can be provided by the neuropsychologist:

Categorization: This section provides information regarding the presence or absence of brain dysfunction and the presence or absence of significant emotional disturbance. The differential diagnosis of a primary organic, a primary functional, or a mixed disorder is made. If significant components of both organic and functional features are present, the relative impact of the two will be discussed.

Localization: Typically, performance of the neuropsychologic test battery can be analyzed to provide data to determine if the brain dysfunction is diffuse or focal. Further analysis provides data regarding the lateralization of the lesion in the right or left hemisphere and localization of the lesion in the anterior or posterior region of the hemisphere. With the advent of new neurodiagnostic procedures (magnetic resonance imaging, positron-emission tomography, and single photon emission computerized tomography [SPECT]), this traditional component of the neuropsychological evaluation has become less important.

Description: Information in this category includes a comprehensive description of the patient's current level of functioning in a wide range of cognitive, adaptive, personality, and behavioral areas. This is perhaps the best usage of neuropsychologic consultation in many cases. The patient's premorbid level of functioning can usually be estimated from the academic and social history and from an analysis of the variability of performance on various tests. From comparisons of the estimated premorbid level of functioning and current performance on standard tests, a relatively accurate indication of deterioration in any of the areas assessed by the battery can be made. A comprehensive overview of the patient's deficits and residual abilities is made, to describe current functioning, explain present behavior, determine the relative effects of organic and functional factors, and provide a baseline of data from which to judge future change. Answers to the question of mental competence and social independence can also be provided by data obtained in the neuropsychologic evaluation.

Prognosis and recommendations: Based on the nature of the neurologic disease and the pattern and degree of deficits seen during the neuropsychologic evaluation, a determination of the probability and degree of expected recovery can be made for many patients. As previously mentioned, a reevaluation some months later greatly aids the ability to make valid prognostic statements in case of either deterioration or recovery. Finally, recommendations for further ancillary evaluations, including psychiatry, speech pathology, occupational therapy, and social service, are made when warranted. Recommendations regarding specific remedial methods or programs may also be made.

Components of the neuropsychologic evaluation: The specific tests used in a neuropsychologic evaluation battery vary with the age of the patient and the nature of the problems, the specific referral questions asked by the physician, and the particular training and experience of the psychologist. Virtually all such test batteries will, however, include assessment of the following functions:

1. History: Developmental, educational, vocational, and social
2. Behavior: Attention, cooperation, level of effort, mood, rapport, and motivation
3. Intelligence: Includes general, verbal, and nonverbal intelligence
4. Language: Includes auditory discrimination, single word and sentence comprehension, repetition, and various aspects of expressive language (e.g., confrontation naming and verbal fluency)
5. Memory: Includes verbal and nonverbal memory, acquisition (new learning), immediate recall, recent and remote memory, incidental memory, and recognition memory
6. Abstract reasoning and executive functions: Includes verbal and nonverbal reasoning, learning to learn, problem solving, and conceptual shifting
7. Spatial analysis and constructional ability: Includes paper-and-pencil reproduction, three-dimensional constructions, reproduction from memory, and visual analysis and organization not requiring a motor response
8. Sensory-perceptual ability: Includes visual, auditory, and tactile perception
9. Geographic orientation
10. Time orientation
11. Achievement in reading, spelling, and calculations
12. Perceptual motor speed: Includes planning ability and concept manipulation
13. Motor strength and coordination
14. Personality
15. Social functioning

From the data generated by the neuropsychologic evaluation, the psychologist typically uses five stages of inference to reach conclusions regarding the patient's neurobehavioral functioning. These include:

1. Levels of performance compared with standard norms (e.g., IQ of 67, with 100 as norm)
2. Levels of present performance compared with known or estimated premorbid levels (e.g., verbal memory quotient of 74 in a practicing lawyer)
3. Variability of performance on tests of different cognitive functions (e.g., verbal scale IQ of 108 [70th percentile] and progressive matrices below the 10th percentile)
4. Discrepancies between tests subsumed by the two hemispheres (e.g., finger-tapping test performance mean of 25 with the right [dominant] hand and 44 with the left hand)
5. Presence of pathognomonic signs (specific behavioral deficits present only with brain dysfunction) (e.g., paraphasic naming errors or unilateral neglect)

References to specific tests that assess these functions and contribute to these inferences are listed in Appendix 1.

In sum, we have found that neurologists and neuropsychologists can beneficially work closely together and make mutually rewarding contributions to the evaluation, description, and management of patients with cognitive and behavioral changes secondary to organic brain disease.

The literature pertaining to clinical neuropsychology has increased almost exponentially since the publication of the first edition of this book. The amount of available material forces the interested reader to be highly selective in choosing books that are both current and clinically pertinent. The state of the art in 1974[32] can now be viewed as an early stage in the proliferation of relevant publications. The following should be considered to be a selective sampling from the available literature: Filskov and Boll,[9,10] Heilman and Valenstein,[12] Horton and Wedding,[13] Lezak,[23] and Kolb and Whishaw.[17]

SPEECH PATHOLOGY

Patients with significant difficulty in communicating should be evaluated by a speech pathologist. All such patients will not be treatment candidates, but, by means of a thorough language evaluation, the speech pathologist is best able to determine appropriate candidates for speech and language therapy and to provide other services to patients who are not selected for treatment. Patients with aphasia, apraxia of speech, and dysarthria are examples of neurologic patients who are appropriate for referral. The speech pathologist should be an important member of any comprehensive rehabilitation team; this is particularly true when a facility sees a large number of stroke patients. Psychogenic speech and language disorders such as elective mutism and hysteric aphonia are ideal conditions for speech evaluation and treatment.

Evaluation by the speech pathologist provides a description of the patient's communicative abilities and deficits, the possible benefits of therapeutic intervention, and a plan for family counseling to facilitate the development of alternative methods of communicating with the patient.

Virtually every physician has access to speech pathologists, either in private practice or in hospital, university, or community clinics. The speech pathologist may be trained at either the master's or the doctoral level. The American Speech and Hearing Association and most states issue licenses or certificates of clinical competence to qualified clinicians. Referring physicians should ensure the basic clinical competence of any speech pathologist they consult. Many speech pathologists will have specialized knowledge and experience in treating patients with articulation disorders, stuttering, or aphasia. The evaluation and treatment of aphasia is a very specialized field, and physicians should determine the speech pathologist's competence in this area before referring such patients to a specific therapist.

Referral

The major reasons for referring patients to a speech pathologist include the following:

1. The mental status examination indicates a communication disorder that requires a more thorough evaluation.
2. An obvious communication disorder exists that requires a screening evaluation to determine the appropriateness of speech therapy.
3. A significant communication disorder is present that requires family counseling to inform the family members about the patient's problem and to assist in maximizing effective communication in the home. This may include alternative modes such as sign language, communication boards, or computer-augmented speech output devices.

The physician may see the following general types of speech and language problems that require more comprehensive evaluation than can be provided in the medical office:

1. Articulation disturbances such as the dysarthrias seen in pseudobulbar palsy, bulbar paralysis, neuromuscular disease such as myasthenia gravis, cerebellar disorders, cerebral palsy, and basal ganglia disease such as parkinsonism
2. Functional (hysteric) aphonias, especially in patients with histories of minor trauma or surgery to the throat or vocal cords
3. Elective mutism
4. Dysfluency (stuttering), which is seen in children and adults; if untreated, may pose a significant obstacle to successful social and vocational adjustment

5. Patients with acquired language disorders (aphasia, alexia, agraphia), deserving an initial speech and language evaluation to determine the potential for speech therapy and to help the patient's family understand and deal with the communication disorder

6. Patients with buccofacial apraxia in the presence or absence of aphasia, who may benefit from speech evaluation and therapy directed toward articulation and the intelligibility of speech, as well as other buccofacial activities such as drinking and swallowing

Speech and Language Evaluation

The comprehensive speech and language evaluation will provide information regarding the following:

Diagnosis: A definition of the primary language disorder (e.g., nonfluent aphasia, dysarthria, buccofacial apraxia).

Description: A comprehensive description of the type of language disorder, including all areas of deficit (e.g., word-finding problems, alexia, or auditory comprehension problems) and residual spared language abilities. The description should contain a quantitative index of the degree of deficit in each area, to allow comparison with subsequent evaluations. Because the patient's functional communicative ability or disability is of primary importance, some statement should be made regarding the effect of the language deficit on the patient's communication ability in formal (test or interview) and informal (social) areas.

Recommendations: Is speech therapy indicated? If so, what will be the emphasis of the therapy? What will be the frequency of therapy visits? What is the projected duration of therapy? What are the specific plans for home therapy by family members and for family counseling? Are communication aids necessary?

Goals of therapy and prognosis: What are the primary goals of speech and language therapy? What is the prognosis for language recovery? What will be the long-term social impact of the language disorder?

Components of the speech and language evaluation: There are numerous systems and methods of speech and language evaluation. The system and the specific tests used will be determined partly by the needs of the particular patient and partly by the individual speech pathologist's training and experience. Because the enumeration of these methods is beyond the scope of this book, the interested reader is referred to Albert and associates,[1] Goodglass and Kaplan,[11] Kertesz,[16] Plum,[30] Porch,[31] Sarno,[34] and Spreen and Risser.[38]

A comprehensive evaluation should include the following elements:

1. An examination of the oral physiology, including the strength and coordination of the muscles of articulation
2. A description of the characteristics of speech articulation—dysarthria, dysfluency, and dysprosody
3. A description of apraxias if present, both verbal (speech) and nonverbal (nonspeech facial movements)
4. An evaluation for aphasia, specifically including an assessment of verbal comprehension, repetition, and word-finding ability, and a description of spontaneous speech
5. An assessment of reading and writing
6. An evaluation of the adequacy of nonverbal communication, including an assessment of the patient's ability to communicate using gestures or other methods regardless of the language deficit
7. A description of the patient's general behavior and specific behavioral responses to the stress of language items

Treatment

Treatment is not universally efficacious in all speech and language disorders.[35] Based on our clinical experience, we have found that, in general, excellent results can often be produced in rehabilitating patients with (1) functional voice disorders, exclusive of elective mutism (which is more resistant to traditional forms of speech therapy); and (2) mild to moderate articulation problems.

Good results can be expected in patients with (1) anomic aphasia, (2) oral apraxia, and (3) moderate articulation problems.

Fair results are generally obtained in patients with (1) Broca's aphasia, (2) moderate to severe articulation problems, (3) aphasia with mild to moderate comprehension defects, and (4) elective mutism (unless intensive, behaviorally oriented therapy is used, in which case the prognosis is improved).

Poor results are typical in therapeutic efforts with patients having (1) global aphasia, (2) Wernicke's aphasia, (3) severe dysarthria and oral apraxia, and (4) language disturbances secondary to dementia.

These are general statements of prognosis; the individual patient with a particular language disorder will not always respond to therapy as projected. Accordingly, a speech and language evaluation of the patient with any developmental or acquired communication disorder is important to provide the opportunity for therapy to those patients who may benefit from it.

PSYCHIATRY

Many patients with organic brain disease will have an associated emotional disturbance that requires psychiatric consultation. Patients referred for psychiatric evaluation include those with psychiatric disorders that preceded their neurologic problem, those with neurologically based emotional problems (e.g., organic mood disorder), those with emotional reactions to brain disease (e.g., reactive depression), those in whom emotional factors complicate dementia, and those with functional disorders that present as neurologic conditions (e.g., hysteric paralysis).[3]

Emotional factors are significant in the rehabilitation and social reintegration of any patient with organic disease. Therefore, a psychiatrist should be consulted to aid in the management of any patient with an emotional problem that is severe enough to interfere with rehabilitative efforts or home adjustment.

There is a resurgence of interest in the subspecialty of neuropsychiatry, and some psychiatrists now have specialized training in organically based behavior changes. The neuropsychiatrist is particularly helpful in working with those patients who are on the borderline between classic neurology and classic psychiatry.

Referral

Because of the relatively high incidence of both mental illness and brain disease, many patients will have coexisting psychiatric and neurologic conditions (e.g., a brain tumor in a schizophrenic patient, a seizure patient with a manic-depressive disorder). For example, we saw a 37-year-old woman with a long psychiatric history. The patient was also an alcoholic and over the years had sustained several significant head injuries. After alcohol withdrawal, she had several grand mal seizures and was admitted to the neurology ward. As her postictal confusion cleared, she demonstrated gross delusional and aggressive behavior. After a complete history taking and medical evaluation, we determined that the patient had an acute neurologic condition superimposed on a preexisting schizophrenia. Because of the significant psychosis, a psychiatrist was consulted for treatment and long-term management.

It is not uncommon for emotionally stable individuals to develop a significant emotional reaction to an acute-onset neurobehavioral disorder such as aphasia. Depressive reactions, anxiety, paranoia, and aggressiveness may develop in response to brain damage. Such emotional reactions may significantly interfere with rehabilitation efforts. For example, a 62-year-old woman developed a right hemiplegia and anomic aphasia secondary to a cerebral thrombosis. After the acute stage, she became increasingly depressed to the point of apathy, self-deprecation, and constant crying. She would no longer actively participate in physical therapy and appeared to abandon any hope of improvement. When a serious emotional reaction such as this is superimposed on an organic deficit, the emotional component must be treated in conjunction with the medical treatment.

Demented patients present a particular challenge because they have both intellectual and emotional changes as a part of the neurologic disease. These changes produce a variety of difficult management problems that are often best handled with the aid of a geriatric psychiatrist or neuropsychiatrist. In the early stage of dementia, patients may retain considerable insight; this capacity to realize the seriousness of their condition often results in profound depression. Other dementing patients are unaware of their deteriorating intellectual ability; such patients often push themselves beyond their capability and thus develop frustration and severe anxiety. For example, a 58-year-old businessman was referred because of failing memory. His examination revealed a genuine memory deficit and other evidence of an early dementia. Severe anxiety was prominent and interfered with both specific test performance and his social and vocational life. This anxiety was greatly reduced by restructuring his lifestyle (e.g., his wife helped him with his business, he discontinued many civic duties, and he used a mild tranquilizer to aid sleep). After several months, retesting showed general cognitive improvement and he was better able to carry out his home and job responsibilities. Anxiety or depression can greatly exacerbate the mental and social disability experienced by the demented patient. The psychiatrist can provide great assistance through the use of psychotropic drugs, family counseling, and general patient management.

The diagnostic problem of differentiating among dementia, depression, and dementia with depression is both common and sometimes difficult in clinical practice. Because this differential diagnosis is critical in terms of patient management and treatment, psychiatrists experienced in dealing with such problems should be involved early in the evaluation process. The misdiagnosis of depression as dementia will deprive the patient of appropriate treatment and leave the family with the erroneous impression that the disease is progressive and irreversible. Conversely, the misdiagnosis of dementia as depression may lead to ineffective and costly psychotherapy, leave the patient subject to the social and vocational problems resulting from intellectual deterioration, and mislead the family as to the prognosis of the disease.

Psychiatric referral is also indicated for patients who develop depression in response to or as a part of a chronic neurologic disease such as myasthenia gravis, epilepsy, multiple sclerosis, amyotrophic lateral sclerosis, or parkinsonism. These patients frequently live long and productive lives if they are able to accept and deal with their disabilities in a realistic fashion.

Many patients with chronic organic mental syndromes such as aphasia, dementia, traumatic encephalopathy, or Korsakoff's disease become management problems and eventually require long-term management in chronic care facilities. Early referral to the psychiatrist or medical social worker can help the family and the physician with the administrative and legal details involved in institutionalization.

A final group of patients who may initially be seen by the neurologist but who require referral to the psychiatrist are patients with somatiform disorders (e.g., hysteric conversion reactions). Such patients will present with symptoms that mimic neurologic disease (e.g., limb paralysis, loss of speech, or sensory loss) but demonstrate no organic etiology after thorough evaluation. The treatment for such functional disorders may be psychotherapy.

Evaluation

The psychiatrist uses psychiatric interview techniques, a psychiatrically oriented mental status examination, and personality tests in the evaluation. Information on specific interview and evaluation techniques is readily available in all major psychiatric texts.[2,14,15,18,20,28,39,40,42]

Treatment

Although specific treatment is frequently unavailable for the primary brain disease, behavioral and pharmacologic treatment can improve the lives of many of these patients.

Medication is particularly useful in patients with preexisting psychiatric disease. In such patients, the underlying psychiatric disorder will respond to a standard regimen of psychotropic medication. Antianxiety or mood-elevating drugs are effective in treating the anxiety or depression frequently seen as a reaction to organic brain disease. Major tranquilizers are often required to control the agitation, delusions, and nocturnal wanderings of the deteriorated organic patient.

Standard psychotherapeutic methods can be used in some organic patients who retain comprehension, memory, and insight. On the other hand, insight therapy would be useless in many patients (e.g., patients with severe amnesia, dementia, significant frontal lobe behavioral changes, and Wernicke's aphasia). In this latter group of patients, behavior modification techniques aimed at specific behaviors are more appropriate and successful.[41]

Family counseling is often the most useful form of patient management. Through discussion, the psychiatrist is able to help the family understand the patient's problem and to offer suggestions on management. With the psychiatrist's help, the family can then restructure the patient's routine in an effort to minimize environmental stress.

The medicolegal aspects of organic disease are also very important and must be part of a long-term management program. The patient's competence to make a will, to conduct personal financial affairs, and to enter into contracts such as marriage should be established in each case.

Finally, every treatment plan should include a consideration of possible eventual full-time supervision if the patient becomes unmanageable in the home. The details of nursing home or institutional placement should be worked out with the help of the psychiatrist, the social worker, and the patient's family. Such plans should be considered early in the course to allow time to assess the family's financial and personal resources; to determine the availability of home nursing services, nursing homes, and institutions; and to preclude the necessity of unsatisfactory and hasty decisions made at a time of crisis.

SOCIAL WORK*

When dealing with neurologic patients and their families in either postacute hospital settings or long-term follow-up and rehabilitation, we have found social workers to be essential resources for better patient management. The primary areas of social work input in such settings include (1) data gathering and evaluation of premorbid, psychosocial, and family information, which is often crucial to understanding the patient and the effect of the neurologic illness or trauma on the patient's ability to function; (2) participation in patient management and family education and support processes during the early recovery stage; and (3) serving as the primary data collator, resource investigator, and coordinator of the referral and placement process when considering and implementing referral to a rehabilitation program or a long-term care facility. Although not all patients and families are in need of all aspects of the social worker's potential role, virtually all can benefit from some component, and many will ultimately require continuing involvement regarding one or more problems of placement, home care services, resource funding, or family education and support.

Virtually all general hospitals, large departments of neurology, and rehabilitation facilities now include social workers as important members of the multidisciplinary team. Hospitals are required to have social service departments and to provide a spectrum of social work services. The clinician in private practice can make use of the staff in the hospital where the patient was admitted, or may make appropriate arrangements for services with community-based private social workers.

Social workers are trained at the undergraduate (BSW) or graduate (MSW, DSW) level; we prefer the higher level of training and clinical experience offered at the graduate level. All states and provinces license or certify social workers with requisite levels of education and experience

* The authors gratefully acknowledge the comments of Callie Black, MSW, BCSW, on an earlier version of this section.

after successful completion of a standard licensing and certifying examination. Additional certification of clinical competence can be obtained from the National Association of Social Workers (ACSW) or the American Board of Examiners in Clinical Social Work (Board Certified Diplomate [BCD]). Both associations publish directories listing qualified members and their areas of particular emphasis. The physician consulting a social worker should ensure that individual's general clinical competence, and especially his or her experience in working with neurologic patients and their families. Social work education and training frequently includes a primary focus such as psychiatric, medical, or community and administrative social work, so individual social workers can vary considerably in terms of their experience and competence in dealing with the neurobehavioral problems and rehabilitation needs of the neurologic patient. We have found medical social workers with broad hospital and clinic experience to work most effectively with our patients.

Consultation

Three groups of patients or families or both most frequently need social work services:

1. Patients who are unable to provide additional information needed by the physician. Family, psychosocial, educational, and vocational data, as well as medical records from previous hospitalizations and treatments performed elsewhere, are frequently most expeditiously gathered by the medical social worker familiar with the physician's needs and the methods of procuring such material. The background information can be collated and presented in an organized fashion to provide a better understanding of the patient and the probable impact of the disease or trauma on his or her future ability to function on a day-to-day basis.
2. Families (and patients) needing information and education, psychologic support, and behavior management techniques to comprehend and deal better with the behavioral and emotional sequelae of neurologic disease.
3. Patients needing referral to comprehensive rehabilitation facilities, long-term care settings, or more focused outpatient therapies. Such plans are often best coordinated with the help of a social worker familiar with community (or regional) resources, funding sources (private insurance carriers, state workman's compensation authorities, and Medicare/Medicaid programs), and the psychologic and logistic needs of the family.

Given the demands of medical practice of rehabilitation facilities, the physician does not usually have sufficient time and knowledge to individually manage these aspects of care and follow-up for each patient. The social worker is uniquely qualified to participate as an integral member of the medical team in this aspect of medical care.

Functions

The specific responsibilities of the social worker typically vary depending on the patient's changing condition and state of hospitalization. The following provides an illustrative outline.

Acute stage: At some point after acute hospitalization the physician may initially consult social service for the purpose of screening for family needs, obtaining family and psychosocial information, or providing direct informational and supportive services to the family. Because of the serious nature of neurologic emergencies, one of the social worker's primary responsibilities is to help the patient's family deal most effectively with the immediate crisis.[6] Moonilal[27] has outlined the primary functions of the social worker during the acute hospital stage as:

1. Informing the patient's family of the patient's condition and the medical procedures in progress, as well as those anticipated for the near future
2. Answering the family's questions and dealing with their immediate concerns; psychologic support is also important at this time
3. Preparing the family for its initial meeting with the patient (after the encounter, families typically have many concerns and questions, and therefore will benefit from further contact with someone who can provide appropriate answers, support, and suggestions)
4. Serving as liaison between family and medical team, a degree of involvement that obviously can work effectively only with the social worker's close and ongoing working relationship with the physicians and nurses providing direct patient care

When the patient is moved to a general medical floor, the social worker frequently remains involved (and may well become more involved) by providing updated information (e.g., translating medical and surgical data into terms that are understandable to the family) and preventing or correcting family misunderstanding of the patient's status and ongoing medical treatment. During this stage, the social worker can also arrange for support and logistic services to meet either the patient's or the family's needs (e.g., transportation, sleeping facilities, financial and legal assistance). Sudden neurologic trauma or illness serves as a significant stressor even to the well-adjusted family. The emotional reaction of family members—especially the spouse of an adult patient and the parents of a patient who is a child—provides an opportunity for direct clinical services in terms of facilitating the expression of normal reactive emotions (grief, depression, anxiety, and anger) and providing support and encouragement directed at helping the family work through such feelings. The recovering patient will require both stability and positive support from family members, so it is important that every effort be made to ensure a realistic family adjustment as the patient moves toward discharge from the acute hospital.

Rehabilitation stage: As the patient moves from the acute hospital stage to the rehabilitation phase, the social worker's role will depend somewhat on the services available at the current hospital. If either a comprehensive rehabilitation program or independent appropriate therapeutic services (e.g., physical, occupational, and speech and language therapy) are offered in the primary hospital, the services offered by the social worker will continue much as they were during the subacute hospital stage. One additional function that may begin at this point is the role as liaison between the rehabilitation team and the family. If it is necessary to arrange for outpatient therapy in another facility or transfer to a specialized rehabilitation program, the social worker typically assumes a primary responsibility for gathering patient hospital data, researching appropriate programs, and coordinating the referral and placement process. A crucial aspect of this process that is well handled by the social worker is researching funding sources for rehabilitation. Although most comprehensive rehabilitation programs maintain a number of "patient recruiters" who aid in the transfer process, such referrals are sufficiently complex that the patient and family benefit from a knowledgeable advocate not directly associated with the facility. The hospital social worker who is familiar with the patient's treatment needs and the family's psychosocial and practical needs can represent their interests when seeking the most appropriate placement.

Hospital discharge: At the time of discharge from the hospital, new fears and crises arise for both patient and family. If discharge results in transfer to the rehabilitation facility, concerns regarding problems at home will be postponed until later. However, efforts should be made to prepare for and prevent any home reintegration problems before they appear. At the time of transfer, the immediate issues involve finding the appropriate placement, arranging the referral and transfer process, and ensuring maximum patient and family acceptance of and initial cooperation with the new facility.

If discharge is to home and family care, both the patient and the family should be prepared for the realities of problems that may arise following transfer from the relatively protective and well-staffed hospital to a home setting. Although the home once may have met all normal needs, the patient's needs are often dramatically changed because of cognitive, sensory-motor, and emotional deficits. The family must now deal with a wide range of problems resulting from the patient's significantly changed status. Family members also will have a variety of anxieties, frustrations, insecurities, and other feelings pertaining both to the realities of the family relationships and to their sometimes inaccurate perceptions of what "should" be done and how it should be carried out.[21]

The social worker is well suited to serve as an extension of the hospital team to the home. Many hospitals include social workers as a part of home health service groups that provide help during this transition period. Patient and family education, psychologic support for all parties, and teaching direct patient management techniques to help the family deal most effectively with any problematic emotional and behavioral changes are only several of the services that can be effective in maximizing the family's positive influence on the patient's recovery. Within this context, the social worker can significantly contribute to positive rehabilitation outcome by:

1. Helping family members to identify and express emotional reactions such as anger, frustration, and sorrow, and to understand that these are natural and expected responses to a highly stressful situation
2. Encouraging family support for the patient's primary caretaker, spouse, and other family members, who will need to recognize their own emotional needs if they are to continue to care effectively for the patient
3. Encouraging the caretaker to rely on his or her own good judgment when conflicts (inevitably) occur with the patient and other family members
4. Facilitating the readjustment of all family members to the necessary new roles and responsibilities
5. Confronting the entire family when divided loyalties are a problem, helping the members to identify and accept their responsibilities, and making necessary changes when the welfare of dependent children is at stake[22]

The effects of neurologic injury or illness are not restricted to the patient alone. Such disorders have an impact on all areas of the patient's life, as well as on family, friends, and fellow workers. Accordingly, efforts must be made to deal with these psychosocial aspects of the problem to try to minimize the negative effects and maximize the social recovery process. Because of their training and experience, the medical social worker can serve as a primary resource for neurologic patients and their families.

COGNITIVE REHABILITATION

Since publication of the first edition of this book, the fields of cognitive retraining and neurorehabilitation have become prominent, albeit somewhat controversial, forces in the treatment of brain-injured patients. Providing specific therapies (e.g., physical, speech-language, psychologic) to promote maximal recovery of particular neurobehavioral deficits after traumatic brain injury or an acute neurologic event (stroke) is not new. However, it has been only in the last 15 to 20 years that comprehensive multidisciplinary team rehabilitation programs have become readily available to such patients. Discussion of the theoretic framework underlying specific cognitive retraining orientations and the nature of comprehensive programs, as well as the practical logistics, advantages, and problems of cognitive rehabilitation programs, is well beyond the focus of this book. The clinician dealing with patients suffering from static neurologic disorders and traumatically induced neurobehavioral deficits should become acquainted with this rapidly evolving area as a potential patient-treatment resource. Decisions regarding whom to refer, when to refer, and particularly where to refer are difficult issues that should be approached with some understanding of the development of this field and an awareness of the positive and negative aspects of particular programs. We suggest Meier, Benton, and Diller;[26] Kreutzer and Wehman;[19] and Rosenthal, Griffith, Bond, and Miller[33] as good introductions to this important field. See especially Lezak[22] for an overview of the assessment process to determine realistic treatment goals and the patient's capability to benefit from rehabilitation.

SUMMARY

The management of patients with organic brain disease is a multidisciplinary effort. Physicians are strongly encouraged to acquaint themselves with the services offered by their colleagues in related specialized fields. With this effort, physicians will be able to better understand their patients and to provide them with more comprehensive care.

REFERENCES

1. Albert, ML, et al: Clinical Aspects of Dysphasia. Springer-Verlag, New York, 1981.
2. American Psychiatric Association: Diagnostic and Statistical Manual of Mental Disorders (DSM-III-R). American Psychiatric Press, Washington, DC, 1987.
3. Benson, DF and Blumer, D (eds.): Psychiatric Aspects of Neurologic Disease, Vol II. Grune & Stratton, New York, 1982.
4. Black, FW: WISC verbal-performance discrepancies as indicators of neurological dysfunction in pediatric patients. J Clin Psychol 30:165, 1974.
5. Black, FW: WAIS verbal-performance discrepancies as predictors of lateralization in patients with discrete missile wounds. Percept Mot Skills 51:213, 1980.
6. Carlton, TO and Stephenson, MDG: Social work and the management of severe head injury. Soc Sci Med 1:5, 1990.
7. Doerr, HO and Carlin, AS: Forensic Neuropsychology. Guilford Press, New York, 1991.
8. Field, J: Two types of tables for use with Wechsler's intelligence scales. J Clin Psychol 16:3, 1960.
9. Filskov, SB and Boll, TJ (eds): Handbook of Clinical Neuropsychology. Wiley-Interscience, New York, 1981.

10. Filskov, SB and Boll, TJ (eds): Handbook of Clinical Neuropsychology, Vol II. Wiley-Interscience, New York, 1986.
11. Goodglass, H and Kaplan, E: The Assessment of Aphasia and Related Disorders, ed 2. Lea & Febiger, Philadelphia, 1983.
12. Heilman, KM and Valenstein, E (eds): Clinical Neuropsychology, ed 2. Oxford University Press, New York, 1984.
13. Horton, AM and Wedding, D: Clinical and Behavioral Neuropsychology. Praeger Scientific Press, New York, 1983.
14. Kaplan, HI and Sadock, BJ: Modern Synopsis of Comprehensive Textbook of Psychiatry II. Williams & Wilkins, Baltimore, 1981.
15. Kaplan, HI and Sadock, BJ: Synopsis of Psychiatry, ed 4. Williams & Wilkins, Baltimore, 1991.
16. Kertesz, A: Aphasia and Associated Disorders: Taxonomy, Localization, and Recovery. Grune & Stratton, New York, 1979.
17. Kolb, B and Whishaw, IQ: Fundamentals of Human Neuropsychology, ed 3. WH Freeman, New York, 1990.
18. Kolb, LC and Brodie, HK: Modern Clinical Psychiatry. WB Saunders, Philadelphia, 1982, pp 184–225.
19. Kreutzer, JS and Wehman, PW: Cognitive rehabilitation for persons with traumatic brain injury. Brookes Publishing, Baltimore, 1991.
20. Lazare, A, Eisenthal, S, and Alonso, A: Clinical evaluation: A multidimensional, hypothesis testing, negotiated approach. In Michaels, R, et al (eds): Psychiatry. JB Lippincott, Philadelphia, 1991, pp 1–13.
21. Lezak, MD: Assessment for rehabilitation planning. In Meier, M, Benton, A and Diller, L (eds): Neuropsychological Rehabilitation. Guilford Press, New York, 1987, pp 41–58.
22. Lezak, MD: Living with the characterologically altered brain injured patient. J Clin Psychol 34:592, 1978.
23. Lezak, MD: Neuropsychological Assessment, ed 2. Oxford University Press, New York, 1983.
24. Matarazzo, JD: Wechsler's Measurement and Appraisal of Adult Intelligence. Williams & Wilkins, Baltimore, 1972.
25. McMahon, EA and Satz, P: Clinical neuropsychology: Some forensic applications. In Filskov, SB and Boll, TJ (eds): Handbook of Clinical Neuropsychology. Wiley-Interscience, New York, 1981, pp 686–701.
26. Meier, M, Benton, A, and Diller, L: Neuropsychological Rehabilitation. Guilford Press, New York, 1987.
27. Moonilal, JM: Trauma centers: A new dimension for hospital social work. Social Work in Health Care 7:15, 1982.
28. Novello, J: The psychiatric history and mental status examination. In Novello, J (ed): A Practical Handbook of Psychiatry. Charles C Thomas, Springfield, IL, 1974, pp 40–48.
29. Parsons, O: Clinical neuropsychology. In Speilberger, C (ed): Current Topics in Clinical Community Psychology, Vol 2. Academic Press, New York, 1970, pp 1–60.
30. Plum, F (ed): Language, Communication, and the Brain. Raven Press, New York, 1988.
31. Porch, B: Porch Index of Communicative Ability. Consulting Psychologists Press, Palo Alto, CA, 1967.
32. Reitan, R and Davison, L (eds): Clinical Neuropsychology: Current Status and Applications. John Wiley & Sons, New York, 1974.
33. Rosenthal, M, et al (eds): Rehabilitation of the adult and child with traumatic brain injury, ed 2. FA Davis, Philadelphia, 1990.
34. Sarno, MT (ed): Acquired Aphasia, ed 2. Academic Press, New York, 1991.
35. Sarno, MT: Recovery and rehabilitation in aphasia. In Sarno, MT (ed): Acquired Aphasia, ed 2. Academic Press, New York, 1991, pp 521–582.

36. Satz, P and Fletcher, JM: Emergent trends in neuropsychology: An overview. J Consult Clin Psychol 49:851, 1981.
37. Spordone, RJ: Neuropsychology for the Attorney. Paul Deutch Press, Orlando, 1991.
38. Spreen, O and Risser, A: Assessment of aphasia. In Sarno, MT (ed): Acquired Aphasia, ed 2. Academic Press, New York, 1991, pp 73–150.
39. Stevenson, I and Sheppe, W: The psychiatric examination. In Arieti, S (ed): The American Handbook of Psychiatry, Vol 1. Basic Books, New York, 1959, pp 215–234.
40. Talbott, JA, Hales, RC, and Yudofsky, SC (eds): Textbook of Psychiatry. American Psychiatric Press. Washington, DC, 1988.
41. Wells, CE and Duncan, GW: Neurology for Psychiatrists. FA Davis, Philadelphia, 1980.
42. Yudofsky, SC and Hales, RE (eds): Textbook of Neuropsychiatry, ed 2. American Psychiatric Press, Washington, DC, 1992.

Appendix 1

Standard Neuropsychologic Tests

The purpose of this section is twofold: (1) to introduce briefly the physician to those tests that are commonly encountered in neuropsychologic reports on patients evaluated because of known or suspected brain dysfunction, and (2) to give the interested psychologist an annotation for those tests and procedures that are representative of those frequently used in neuropsychology or that have proved their clinical utility to the authors. It is not intended as a comprehensive overview of neuropsychologic procedures nor as an in-depth evaluation of any individual technique. See Lezak[76] or Spreen and Strauss[114] for such presentations.

SCREENING TESTS

Clinical psychologists who wish to screen briefly for the possibility of neurologic problems during a routine assessment should include one of the following tests in their evaluation: (1) The Neuropsychological Screening Exam[93] is a psychometrically oriented mental status examination that evaluates a number of neurobehavioral functions in a brief (40 to 60 minutes) period, yielding a "cutting" score to estimate the probability of dysfunction. In contrast, (2) the Adult Neuropsychological Questionnaire[85] and (3) the Neuropsychological Status Examination[94] consist of structured interviews to collect historic and current complaint data that can be used to suggest the presence of problems requiring more extensive evaluation. (4) The Neuropsychological Impairment Scale[88-90] is a 50-item self-report screening test designed to identify neuropsychologic symptoms and deficits. Preliminary research[88,89] suggests that it is reasonably sensitive, valid, and reliable when used for its stated purpose—brief screening. (5) The Luria-Nebraska Neuropsychological Battery (LNNB)[41] contains a 34-item "pathognomic scale" that has shown some efficacy in differentiating between patients with organic and nonorganic disease.[128] (6) The Screening Test for the LNNB[38] purports to predict overall LNNB scores accurately, using a 20-minute procedure. Although this method may have some appeal to clinicians comfortable with the LNNB, research results have been insufficient to recommend its use as a general screen for neurobehavioral dysfunction. Other clinical researchers have devised a variety of screening batteries based on a number of relatively brief measures derived from the Halstead-Reitan Battery and other sources. See Berg, Franzen, and Wedding[15] for further information regarding such screening procedures.

None of these tests and methods is capable of doing more than increasing the suspicion of neurobehavioral dysfunction. They do not replace the need for doing more comprehensive testing when indicated; they do not unequivocally identify brain-damaged patients; and they cannot provide the data necessary for an accurate and detailed description of the patient's present neuropsychologic status. As screening techniques, they can be used with some utility if properly employed by an experienced clinician.

COMPREHENSIVE NEUROPSYCHOLOGIC BATTERIES

Halstead-Reitan Battery

This battery includes a well-standardized series of tests of cognitive and adaptive ability. It was originally introduced by Halstead,[51] revised and standardized by Reitan and associates,[17,30,33,100,102,117] and statistically refined by Russell and associates[105] and others.[117] A recent publication[56] has provided significantly improved age-graded norms for the basic Halstead-Reitan battery and for many additional tests frequently used in association with this battery. The primary limitations of this battery include its length, the minimal emphasis of the battery on important neurobehavioral areas such as memory and language, and a lack of data results that can be readily translated to functionally relevant descriptive information for the nonneuropsychologist. Its primary approach, which is the diagnosis of brain dysfunction and not the delineation and description of functional disabilities, appears somewhat dated in an era of magnetic resonance imaging (MRI) for anatomic visualization and positron-emission tomography (PET) to assess physiologic functioning of the brain. However, augmented by the addition of tests of general cognitive ability, language, and memory, this battery is currently one of the best and most popular standardized methods of identifying patients with neurologic dysfunction.[76]

Luria's Neuropsychologic Investigation

Christensen[22] organized some of Luria's materials and techniques into a written format, with a manual of administration instructions, in a framework that corresponded to his conceptualization of brain function-behavior relationships. This contribution allows the well-trained clinician to use and adapt Luria's experimental procedures for patient examination. The battery includes techniques that assess math functions, auditory-motor organization, kinesthetic functions, higher visual functions, receptive and expressive language, reading and writing, arithmetic skill, memory, and intellectual processes. It is limited in the testing of attention and vigilance, visual memory, and nonverbal abstract reasoning. Its advantage is its ready adaptability to meet the needs of each individual case. However, its lack of normative data restricts the interpretation of some items to a very well-trained and highly experienced examiner. The use of Christensen's materials and especially Luria's approach and techniques cannot be considered a ready-to-use test in the sense of psychometrically based approaches to neuropsychologic assessment. Although very interesting and often useful in providing detailed information about the individual patient, any clinician interested in this approach must be thoroughly versed in Luria's philosophy, theories, and techniques and be prepared to design single-subject experimental investigations for each patient.

Luria-Nebraska Neuropsychological Battery

This battery,[39-41] which is an attempt to standardize and provide normative data on selected items adapted from the Christensen-Luria materials, has been the source of both considerable clinical popularity and major criticism in the neuropsychologic literature since its inception. Golden and colleagues[39,40] have consistently reported the battery's ability to differentiate brain-damaged patients from normal people and psychiatric patients, whereas others have concluded that the battery is not diagnostically reliable.[1,26] Reviews of the positive and negative findings with the LNNB can be found in Spiers[111] and Stambrook.[115] At the time of the second edition of this book, the LNNB was viewed by most neuropsychologists as a battery with some potential—not yet realized—as a comprehensive neuropsychologic instrument. To date, this status has not changed. The battery now seems less popular than at the time of previous editions of this book.[20]

TESTS OF GENERAL COGNITIVE FUNCTIONING

Wechsler Adult Intelligence Scale–Revised

The Wechsler Adult Intelligence Scale–Revised (WAIS-R)[125] is the current revision and standardization of the adult Wechsler Scales. The test, which remains the standard for the clinical assessment of intelligence for patients between 16 and 74 years of age, provides data that reflect general intellectual functioning (full-scale IQ), verbal and nonverbal performance (verbal and performance scale IQs), and specific subtest performance in the following areas:

VERBAL SCALE	PERFORMANCE SCALE
Information	Picture completion
Digit span	Picture arrangement
Vocabulary	Block designs
Arithmetic	Object assembly
Comprehension	Digit symbol
Similarities	

The summary IQ scores derived from the WAIS-R (and most other commonly used intelligence tests) have a normative mean of 100, with a standard deviation of 15.

Use of the WAIS-R with neurologic patients allows an analysis of performance at several levels of inference that are valuable in neuropsychologic assessment: comparisons of an individual patient's performance with that of normative and clinical samples, comparisons of current performance with either estimated or documented premorbid functioning, and analyses of intraindividual performance on subtests that assess different areas of cognitive functioning (e.g., verbal versus nonverbal or verbal-comprehension versus perceptual-analytic versus attention-concentration).[109] A Spanish language version of the test, which was standardized in Puerto Rico, is available,[47] as is the Wechsler Intelligence Scale for Children—III,[123] for use with patients under age 16. Edith Kaplan has recently introduced the "WAIS-R as a Neuropsychological Instrument,"[61] which represents a synthesis of the process-oriented approach to the neuropsychologic analysis of general cognitive functioning. After administration of the standard WAIS-R, this technique provides additional subtests, an alternate multiple-choice format for further assessment of the pattern and style of patients' functioning on a number of the subtests, a more comprehensive method of assessing specific deficits in arithmetic, and a new symbol copy task to better delineate the visuospatial processes involved in the standard Digit Symbol subtest.

The WAIS-R (and previously the WAIS and Wechsler-Bellevue) has served as an essential component of virtually all standard neuropsychologic evaluations. The additions provided by the Kaplan method of administration and interpretation should result in even more valuable information from this test. More comprehensive reviews of the neuropsychologic use of the Wechsler Scales may be found in Golden and Vicente;[42] Matarazzo;[82] Lezak;[76] Lawson, Inglis, and Stroud,[69] and Kaplan.[61]

Leiter International Performance Scale

The Leiter International Performance Scale (LIPS) is a measure of intelligence that uses a picture stimulus-block matching paradigm for use with nonverbal children and adults.[70,71] The test consists of a graduated series of subtests, ranging from simple matching of color, shape, and number to more complex relationships of design patterns and visual analogies. At its upper levels, reasonably complex problem solving is required. A detailed manual covering test administration, scoring, and interpretation is available, which also gives a summary of research studies and basic normative information.[74] Although not well standardized in terms of gradation of item difficulty, validity, and reliability at the higher levels (ages 14 to adult), it is a useful adjunct in those situations when a purely nonverbal test is needed. The primary advantage of this test is that it requires no verbal response from the patient and little or no verbal input on the examiner's part, making it appropriate for use with auditorily handicapped, non-English-speaking, and educationally deprived patients.

Stanford-Binet, Fourth Edition

The Stanford-Binet test, fourth edition,[119] is an age-graded, moderately verbally loaded test of general intelligence, which includes 15 subtests arranged in order of difficulty (and, ostensibly, of mental age). The test provides standard age scores (generally compatible with intelligence summary scores) with a mean of 100 and a standard deviation of 16 in the areas of verbal reasoning, abstract and visual reasoning, quantitative reasoning, and short-term memory. There is also an overall index of functioning, the test composite standard age score, which is akin to a full-scale IQ. It can be used with patients from age 2 through adulthood. Originally designed primarily for use with children, it is not used as a part of most standard neuropsychologic batteries. However, it is useful in situations when the WAIS-R cannot or should not be administered for any reason. The previous editions of the Stanford-Binet test had the disadvantage of being very global in nature, with only an overall IQ being obtained. This problem has been resolved to some degree in the fourth edition, with the four factor scores appearing to have sufficient statistical robustness to allow pattern analysis. Currently, its primary applications for the neuropsychologist are in dealing with very low-functioning adult patients who do not have language dysfunction, and when a general intellectual reevaluation is required and the WAIS-R is not appropriate (e.g., when test-retest practice effects would be problematic). The revised Stanford-Binet test is a dramatic improvement over its previous edition and is now at least a feasible alternative to the WAIS-R for use in neuropsychologic assessment, although it cannot be considered an equivalent measure.

MEASURES OF PREMORBID FUNCTIONING

Interpretation of the clinical significance of neuropsychologic findings of the individual patient is partly dependent on changes in functioning from premorbid levels. This is true in medicolegal, clinical, and research situations.[81] If they can be obtained without undue problem, premorbid school records frequently contain the results of group tests of general ability (e.g., Otis-Lenon Test, Scholastic Aptitude Test, and the like), which are useful for comparison purposes. Reports of school grades may also be used. However, such records do not provide data comparable to the results obtained from the neuropsychologic evaluation, except in very broad terms. A number of techniques for estimating premorbid intellectual functioning from data and/or information gathered during the neuropsychologic evaluation have been devised, including use of the WAIS-R subtests of Vocabulary and Information, performance on tests of reading recognition (especially the National Adult Reading Test),[106] reliance on the patient's highest level of functioning on any test or set of tests, and the development of statistic regression equations based on demographic information. See Lezak[76] and Spreen and Strauss[114] for further descriptions of these techniques.

The use of demographic variables to predict premorbid intelligence statistically has the advantages of using data readily generated during the neuropsychologic evaluation, applying equally to virtually all patients, and not declining because of a clinical condition.[114] Barona, Reynolds, and Chastain[7] have developed and refined a regression equation for predicting WAIS-R Verbal, Performance, and full-scale IQs using the variables of age, sex, race, educational level, occupation, urban-rural residence, and geographic region of birth. The method appears to provide reasonably valid estimates of premorbid functioning within the IQ range between 69 and 120.

TESTS OF ATTENTION AND VIGILANCE

Digit Repetition

The number of digits repeated *forward* on the WAIS-R or any other string of single-digit numbers provides an easily administered objective measure of the patient's ability to maintain auditory attention for a brief period (approximately 10 to 15 seconds). The WAIS (but not the WAIS-R) manual provides a method of converting raw digit-repetition scores to standard scores. Note that both administration and scoring of the Digit Scan subtest have been changed for the WAIS-R, making it a somewhat different task neuropsychologically. Digit span repeated *backward* requires different mental processes, and cognitively differs appreciably from digits repeated forward. Although attention is certainly *one* of the requirements of this task, it is far from the primary component of such performance.

"A" Random Letter Test for Vigilance

This test is well described in Chapter 4. In addition to its use in the mental status examination, we have devised a longer version of the test for tape presentation. This test consists of a 5-minute string of random letters presented at a rate of 1 per second, with the patient asked to signify by raising his or her finger (or by whatever means possible) whenever the letter "A" is heard. The series of A's includes several runs of four, three, and two sequential presentations of the target letter, to assess the patient's ability to inhibit an ongoing response pattern or tendency to perseverate. The test is scored for omission, commission, and perseverative errors; average individuals are able to perform without error (or at the most, with an error due to boredom). The advantages of this form of the test are that it demands a greater degree of effort and measures sustained attention or vigilance for a more functionally meaningful period of time.

Letter and Symbol Cancellation Tasks

A variety of visually presented letter, number, and symbol cancellation tasks are available to evaluate the patient's ability to maintain visual attention for varying periods. They typically include an array of randomly presented visual stimuli with a given target item that must be noted and crossed out. They range from the relatively straightforward (six rows of 52 characters, with the target letter appearing approximately 18 times)[29] to the highly complex (two pages containing 25 rows of 30 randomly distributed digits, with the target digit changing with each line.[87] The arrays presented by Mesulam[86,86a] are particularly useful, as their format allows the examiner to detect unilateral neglect and inattention as well as the patient's vigilance. See Lezak[76] for an overview of these methods.

Paced Auditory Serial Addition Test

The Paced Auditory Serial Addition Test (PASAT)[49] is a highly demanding and sensitive test of active verbal attention, information processing, and basic ability to calculate. It consists of a taped presentation of 60 pairs of randomized digits, with the requirement that each digit is added to the previously presented digit (e.g., for the presented numbers "3-6-2-9-8," the correct response would be "9-8-11-17"). The digits are presented at four different rates of speed, ranging from one digit every 1.2 second to one every 2.4 seconds. Derived scores include the percentage of correct responses at each rate or the mean score. Additional age-graded norms have been recently published, extending the clinical utility of this test.[104] The PASAT has been used with a wide range of neurologic conditions, and frequently appears in the research literature pertaining to the behavioral effects and recovery from mild and moderate closed head injury.[72,73] See Gronwall[48] for a recent review of this technique.

TESTS OF LANGUAGE FUNCTIONING

Peabody Picture Vocabulary Test–Revised

The Peabody Picture Vocabulary Test–Revised (PPVT-R) is an easily administered test of single-word vocabulary comprehension. It includes two equivalent sets of stimuli plates, each of which contains four pictures. The two individual word lists include 175 words in ascending order of difficulty. The patient indicates which of the four pictures represents the word provided by the examiner (e.g., "Where is 'exhausted'?"). Norms are provided for age groups between 2½ and 41 years. The test is useful for many reasons: (1) It serves as a useful "icebreaker," as its graded format allows absolute success at some level; (2) it provides an assessment of the patient's ability to understand spoken language at its basic (one-word) level; and (3) it gives a general approximation of the patient's level of intellectual functioning because of the relatively high correlation between the PPVT-R and standard adult intelligence tests (0.65 to 0.75). It should be emphasized that this is *not* a test of intelligence; neither current nor premorbid IQ estimates should be made based on Peabody test performance. Its primary use is in providing an objective test of single-word receptive vocabulary, with an important secondary goal of providing the psychologist with an early estimation of the patient's probable ability to perform on the language-mediated elements of the neuropsychologic evaluation.

Token Test

The short version of the Token Test[28] is a well-structured, simply administered test of language comprehension, which assesses an ability to respond to various sentence types, semantic relations, and linguistic elements. It uses colored plastic tokens that are manipulated by the patient in response to a series of hierarchically ordered verbal commands (e.g., from "show me a circle" to "after touching the yellow circle, pick up the white square"). It is useful in the assessment of aphasic patients, as well as those with comprehension deficits secondary to dementia, other neurologic conditions, or low levels of general intelligence. A number of versions of the Token Test have been devised and are well reviewed in Lezak.[76]

Boston Naming Test

The Boston Naming Test (BNT)[62] is a measure of visual confrontation naming. A verbal production reciprocal of the PPVT-R, it requires the patient to name a 60-item series of pictured objects ordered in increasing difficulty from "bed" to "abacus." If the patient is unable to spontaneously name an item, the examiner provides first a categoric cue (e.g., "it's something to eat") and then a phonemic one (e.g., the beginning sound of the target word). The test is basically a test of single-word expressive vocabulary or naming ability. Provisional norms are provided in the manual for children, normal adults, and aphasic adults, with additional norms derived from both normal and clinical samples being readily available.[114] In addition to a comparison of the patient's general level of functioning with normative data, the frequency and type of paraphasic naming errors can be readily determined. Because of the frequent incidence of naming problems in a wide range of clinical conditions, and the ease of administration of the test, the BNT has deservedly become a very popular measure.

Verbal Fluency Tests

A number of standardized tests of verbal fluency are currently available. The two that have proved most effective in our setting are the Controlled Oral Word-Association Test (FAS or CFL), adopted from the Multilingual Aphasia Examination (MAE),[12] and the Animal-Naming Test, adopted from the Boston Diagnostic Aphasia Examination (BDAE).[43] These tests are discussed in Chapter 5. Both objectively measure the patient's ability to produce spontaneously words under the restrictions of a limited category (e.g., "F") and time (60 seconds). Spreen and Strauss[114] provide an update of normative data for these tests.

Analogs of this verbal task are available for written language[118] and reading.[8]

Sentence Repetition

The two widely used tests of sentence repetition are the Spreen-Benton Sentence Repetition Test[112] and Sentence Repetition from the Multilingual Aphasia Examination.[12] Both tests assess the patient's ability to repeat immediately a series of sentences of increasing length and semantic complexity. Given the nature of this method, both verbal memory (immediate recall) and linguistic functioning must be considered in the interpretation of deficient repetition. Measures of repetition are most frequently used with patients having a known aphasia, with transcortical and conduction aphasics providing the most striking results. Norms are available for both normal and neurologically impaired adults, as well as for children.

Comprehensive Aphasia Batteries

When evaluating a patient with known aphasia or a clinically apparent language obstacle to valid neuropsychologic evaluation, a complete aphasia examination should be conducted. In some settings, this is the responsibility of the speech pathologist; in other settings, such batteries are used by the neuropsychologist. In either case, the clinician who deals with brain-damaged patients should be familiar with the contents as well as the advantages and disadvantages of the commonly used measures. The following is an annotated listing of the more popular batteries; the reader is referred to Albert and associates,[4] Lezak,[76] Kertesz,[64] and Spreen and Strauss[114] for more thorough reviews of the evaluation process in aphasia, as well as for reviews of the specific tests.

Test batteries are listed in alphabetic order. Our preference is for the BDAE or the similar Western Aphasia Battery, although each of the listed tests has enjoyed considerable popularity.

Aphasia Language Performance Scales

This is a short (30-minute) test[63] of communicative ability designed primarily to determine the suitability of the patient for speech and language therapy.

Boston Diagnostic Aphasia Examination

This highly clinical battery, now in its second edition,[44] systematically assesses virtually all areas of language. The test is useful for the description of aphasic disorders, treatment planning, and research.

Communication Abilities in Daily Living

Communication Abilities in Daily Living (CADL) is a test[57] of functional daily communication ability in aphasic adults, which is primarily used by speech therapists to determine those aspects of communication that should be treated to maximize functional communication. Because of its emphasis on the patient's ability to communicate using any means, including gestures, writing, pointing, and the like, the CADL is a good adjunct to other language assessment methods, which concentrate on the accuracy of language performance.

Multilingual Aphasia Examination

The MAE[12] is a research-derived systematic examination of the major components of speech and language. Each scale is objectively and independently scored, allowing independent use of subtests. The examination is neuropsychologically oriented and appropriate for research.

Neurosensory Center Comprehensive Examination for Aphasia

The Neurosensory Center Comprehensive Examination for Aphasia (NCCEA)[113] is a comprehensive battery that assesses 20 different components of language. It also includes four tests of tactile and visual functioning. Because of the nature of its content, it is useful for neurolinguistic research but suffers somewhat when used clinically with patients having only a mild degree of aphasia. A recent updating of normative data is now available.[114]

Porch Index of Communicative Ability

The Porch Index of Communicative Ability (PICA)[91] is a highly structured, standardized, psychometrically oriented battery that is used to quantify a variety of communicative functions, including verbal, gestural, and graphic. The test is most frequently used by speech pathologists to establish baseline levels, predict probable recovery, and quantify the results of therapy and spontaneous improvement. Its statistical sophistication allows certain types of research; however, because it is psychometrically and not clinically oriented, it is not especially useful in the neurobehavioral study of the classic aphasic syndromes.

Western Aphasia Battery

This battery[65] is essentially an adaptation and standardization of the BDAE, incorporating many of the same items and using the same theoretic framework for classification of aphasic subtypes. It includes tests of constructional ability, arithmetic, praxis, and Raven's Matrices to assess functions related to communication. The test has become relatively popular, perhaps because of its psychometric properties. Its clinical and research utility does not differ significantly from that of the more established BDAE. It is of incidental interest that the Western Aphasia Battery was designed for and standardized on Canadians.

TESTS OF MEMORY

Wechsler Memory Scale–Revised

The publication of the Wechsler Memory Scale–Revised (WMS-R)[124] in 1987 provided neuropsychologists with a major new omnibus measure of memory functioning. The WMS-R represents a significant improvement over the memory tests previously available, although a number of reviews of its composition and psychometric properties[18,32,78] rather strongly suggest that it is not the ideal test that had been hoped for. Notwithstanding its limitations, the WMS-R has become the most frequently administered comprehensive measure of memory performance. It provides summary scores for general, verbal, visual, and delayed memory, and a measure of attention and concentration. Specific functioning is evaluated in the verbal areas of logical paragraph recall (immediate and after a 30-minute delay) and verbal paired associate learning (immediate and delayed); the visual areas of figural memory, visual paired learning (immediate and delayed), and visual design reproduction (immediate and delayed); and the attention-concentration areas of mental control, digit span, and visual memory span (a visually presented analog of digit repetition). The WMS-R is rather well standardized, with normative data provided for age groups between 16 and 74. Golden[37] gives a recent overview of the clinical use of the WMS-R, with comments regarding its advantages and disadvantages.

Rey Auditory Verbal Learning Test

The Rey Auditory Verbal Learning Test (RAVLT)[103] is an easily administered test of immediate verbal memory span. In five acquisition trials of a 15-word list, the test provides a learning curve and documents learning strategies (primacy or recency effects), retroactive and proactive interference, and intrusion errors, confusion, or confabulation tendencies. An interference trial followed by an immediate recall of the acquisition list and a short-term recall after a 20-minute time delay provide retention scores. Recognition memory is assessed after the delayed recall trial. With additional delayed trials (60 minutes, 24 hours, and so forth), the test can also measure retention over time. Rey[103] and others have provided an objective scoring method and normative data for acquisition, recall after interference, delayed recall, and recognition trials, drawn from normal and clinical samples. A nonverbal analog of this test in picture form[33] has also been studied. This test is not widely used in clinical batteries, but it would seem to be useful in assessing patients with memory disorders, in investigating cognitive function in patients with unilateral hemispheric lesions, or in the experimental study of memory.

California Verbal Learning Test

The California Verbal Learning Test (CVLT)[27] uses the same list learning format as other verbal learning tests but offers the advantage of using a word list that can be encoded by several different methods. This allows the examiner to assess learning and memory by measuring coding strategies, learning rates, other process data, and short- and long-term delay. The test manual gives preliminary normative data for seven age groups, ranging from 17 to 80 years. Because of the popularity of this measure, a wise range of data is now available from a variety of clinical and experimental groups. The CVLT is a robust test of verbal list learning and recall that has sufficient advantage over similar measures that it is probably preferable.

Randt Memory Test

Randt and colleagues[19,95,96] designed a brief (20- to 30-minute) test battery to assess objectively memory acquisition, storage, and retrieval.

The test is theoretically and psychometrically superior to other clinical memory batteries and has the added value of a 24-hour delayed recall. It shares the WMS's verbal emphasis, with disproportionately fewer sensitive measures of nonverbal memory. Early clinical and experimental work suggested that the Randt test could become a useful component of the neuropsychologic evaluation. Despite some recent studies,[34] however, the test has not attained the degree of usage necessary to generate normative and clinical data sufficient to allow its development beyond the stage of an interesting experimental procedure. It has now been largely overshadowed by the WMS-R and other more recent comprehensive memory batteries, although its formative data for 24-hour recall can be useful in certain cases.

Memory Assessment Scales

The Memory Assessment Scales (MAS)[126] is the most recently published comprehensive battery for assessing memory functioning in adults. It includes 12 subtests, based on seven learning and recall tasks, and provides summary scores for short-term memory (verbal span and visual span), verbal memory (word list recall and immediate recall of a logical paragraph), visual reproduction (15-second recall of visual designs and immediate visual recognition of visual designs), and global memory. There are additional verbal process scores and scores reflecting intrusion errors, clustering of responses during acquisition and recall tasks, performance after cues, and recognition memory. A clinically and experimentally interesting name-face auditory-visual paired associate learning subtest is included, although it is not included in the computation of summary memory scores.

The MAS manual includes norms based on 843 adults, aged 18 to 90. Separate tables are provided (1) by age decade, (2) by age and educational level, and (3) for 467 adults selected to match the US census on the basis of age, education, and gender. Preliminary use of the MAS suggests that it should be quite useful in both clinical and research settings. Because it is new, however, relatively few studies have been published regarding its use, and there are few data comparing it to the more widely distributed WMS-R.

Bender's Gestalt Incidental Recall

Incidental visual memory may be assessed by requesting the patient to recall and produce the nine Bender Gestalt designs shortly after completion of the reproduction phase of the test. In contrast to most memory tests, the patient is not told that he or she will be required to recall the designs, thus eliminating the concentration and practice effects that occur when the patient is aware of the "memory" nature of the test. In initial attempts to standardize this procedure and from considerable clinical use, we have found that normal subjects correctly recall a mean of six designs (standard deviation of approximately 1). It has been useful in demonstrating defects in patients who perform relatively adequately on the Memory for Designs (MFD) (farther on) or the Benton Visual Retention Test (BVRT) when they know that they must make a concentrated effort to remember.

Benton Visual Retention Test

The BVRT[11] consists of several series of simple and complex line drawings that are presented to the patient for varying periods (5 to 10 seconds, depending on the administration form). The patient reproduces the designs directly or does so after a variable delay (immediate recall or a 15-second delay). This test, which was designed to assess visual perception and analysis, short-term visual memory, and constructional ability, has explicit scoring instructions and robust normative data. It is useful with a wide age range and has repeatedly proved effective in clinical situations.[80]

Memory for Designs

The MFD[46] consists of 15 line drawings of variable complexity that are displayed to the patient one at a time for 5 seconds each. Immediately after termination of exposure, the patient reproduces the design. An objective scoring system is provided, but the procedures contain questionable methods (e.g., totally forgotten designs are not considered, and there is an overemphasis on rotated or reversed reproductions), thus reducing the clinical utility of the tests. Studies of the efficacy of the MFD to detect brain-damaged patients do not generally support its usefulness when compared with similar tests.[55] Accordingly, although this test remains popular with many clinicians, the BVRT is preferred.

Recurring Figures Test

This test, designed by Kimura,[66] assesses visual recognition memory and rate of forgetting. The patient is initially presented with a set of 20 geometric and irregularly drawn nonsense figures that include eight stimulus designs. The patient is then shown a pack of 140 designs composed of seven sets of the original eight designs interspersed with 84 unique designs. The patient is asked to indicate whenever a previously seen design is shown. Scores that reflect total correct responses and total correct geometric versus nonsense designs are obtained, as well as a curve of "forgetting" over the seven trials. The test has been used clinically to differentiate brain-damaged patients from normal patients and to lateralize lesions, and in experimental studies of memory processing.[67]

Tactual Performance Test

Reitan[100] incorporated the Tactual Performance Test (TPT) as a core measure in his battery. It had initially been adapted by Halstead from Sequin's original 10-piece wooden form board. The TPT requires the blindfolded patient to complete the form board first using the dominant hand only, then using the nondominant hand only, and finally using both hands. After completion of the three trials, all test items and the blindfold are removed, and the patient is instructed to draw a picture of the form board with shapes correctly aligned. Scores are obtained for the time required to complete each trial, for each correct shape remembered during the drawing trial, and for each correctly positioned drawn shape. The presumption in the use of this test is that learning takes place over the three direct trials and that nonverbal memory is tapped during the recall phase. Despite its continuing popularity as a part of the Halstead-Reitan battery, there are many reservations regarding its utility, including the neuropsychologically complex nature of the tasks, the time necessary for administration, and the tremendous discomfort and frustration experienced by many patients. The test does not currently seem cost effective in terms of any unique data that it might provide.

TESTS OF ABSTRACTION AND HIGHER COGNITIVE FUNCTION

Shipley-Hartford Scale

The Shipley-Hartford Scale[108] is a measure of verbal logical reasoning, in which performance on a subtest of verbal abstract reasoning presented as a series of incomplete progressions (e.g., up-down, in-out, come-_____) is contrasted with a baseline derived from a multiple-choice vocabulary test. The rationale for this test is that with many organic deficits, vocabulary will usually be better retained, whereas abstraction and intellectual efficiency will show greater impairment. A recent revised scoring system and additional normative data are now available.[129] Swiercinsky[117] suggested, on the basis of a factor analytic study, that the Shipley-Hartford scale was a time-effective, cost-effective, and clinically appropriate substitute for the much more time-consuming Category Test for assessing abstraction. Although this is probably not a wise substitution, the test can be useful in assessing verbal abstract reasoning in some situations. The Shipley-Hartford Scale's reliance on written verbal stimuli limits its use in general neuropsychologic practice to cases in which normal language functioning and a reading level at approximately the eighth-grade level have been established.

Wisconsin Card-Sorting Test

The Wisconsin Card-Sorting Test (WCST),[14] which was designed to assess abstract ability, conceptual set shifting, and "learning to learn" using tasks of medium-level complexity, was revised in terms of administration and scoring directions and has been subjected to a more refined standardization study.[54] In this test the patient must sort a series of printed cards according to color, form, or number, with the corrected category shifting without notice each time the criterion of 10 consecutive correct responses is reached. The patient is told whether a response is right or wrong but is not informed that the category will shift or what the correct category is. This test has received renewed neuropsychologic attention because (1) it provides an objective measure of abstraction and problem solving; (2) it has been purported to be sensitive differentially to the effects of frontal lobe lesions (although this has not been consistently found); and (3) it gives information on the particular reasons for difficulty on the test (e.g., impaired conceptualization, failure to sustain the correct set, perseveration, or deficits in learning across several trials). WCST scores usually reported include the number of categories (correct sorts) attained, ranging from 0, when the patient is never able to reach the criterion of 10 sequential correct responses when sorting to color, to 6, when the test is typically discontinued; the number or percentage of perseverative errors; the number of trials required to complete the first category; and the number of "failure to maintain set" errors, which reflects the patient's inability to maintain usage of a successful sorting strategy. Computer scoring of test protocols and an experimental computer administration of the WCST are now available. As with the Category Test, results obtained on the WCST may be confounded by the effects of general intelligence and academics, thus requiring careful interpretation in the individual patient.

Category Test

Many consider the Category Test[101] to be among the most sensitive tests of the Halstead-Reitan battery to the effects of brain dysfunction. Administered with a slide projector, it measures abstract reasoning and problem solving, with tasks of moderate-level complexity. The patient is required to learn sorting behavior based on such variables as size, shape, number, color, position, and brightness. Category Test performance has been demonstrated to be related to age, education, and intelligence, resulting in interpretation problems when evaluating the performance of some patients. We have also noted problems caused by the effects of variable attention and effort. Reliance on the standard absolute error score cutoff as suggested by Reitan is probably unwise. However, newer, age-based norms[56] have proved helpful and should be used when this test is given. The Category Test in its standard form is expensive, time-consuming, and frustrating to many patients. These logistical problems, combined with the psychologic complexity of the test and the complex nature of the derived test score, raise questions as to the cost- and time-effectiveness of this widely used instrument, as well as its validity and utility in some cases. In efforts to deal with at least the cost and logistics problems, both short forms[21] and paper-and-pencil forms[2,24] of the test have been developed. We have found the Booklet Category Test[25] to be a useful measure of higher-order conceptual functioning, and it is certainly more easily transported and administered in a hospital setting.

Raven's Progressive Matrices

Raven's Progressive Matrices[97-99] is a test of visuospatial analysis, spatial conceptualization, and numerical reasoning. The test is available in three difficulty levels, ranging from the Coloured Matrices for children and impaired adults to the Advanced Matrices for well-functioning adults. It is easily administered, taking from 15 to 30 minutes, and requires the patient to select a pictured pattern from a series of alternative possibilities to best complete a stimulus pattern with an omitted portion. The matrices are useful for assessing visual pattern analysis, matching, nonverbal reasoning, unilateral neglect, and cognitive style.

In patients with known perceptuomotor or constructional deficits, the test can be useful for differentiating between the visuospatial analytic and the motor-integration components of the problem. In brain-damaged patients, the degree of impairment seems directly related to the extent of damage, with a tendency for right hemisphere–damaged patients to perform less adequately, especially on the colored version of the test.[101]

Proverbs Test

A variety of proverb interpretation tests have been devised to assess the patient's level of abstract versus concrete thinking. Verbal abstraction should be considered to be a continuum, ranging from complete abstract thinking to absolute concreteness. Accordingly, the response to proverbs should not be interpreted in a dichotomous fashion (concrete-abstract) but rather by rating the adequacy of an answer on a scale (e.g., 1, 2, 3, 4, 5) that objectifies the degree of abstract ability. The Proverbs Test[45] is a standardized test of proverb interpretation, with items presented at variable levels of familiarity and difficulty. The patient is presented with four alternative interpretations for each proverb, one of which is the correct abstract response; one of which is a literal, concrete interpretation; and two of which are either of variable levels of inaccuracy or are common misinterpretations. The structured multiple-choice format of the test has the advantage of providing objective scores of both abstraction and concreteness that can be compared with standard norms. It does not allow the total inadequacy of interpretation or the variety of concrete responses that are produced by some patients on less-structured versions of the task.

TESTS OF SENSORY-PERCEPTUAL FUNCTIONING

Seashore Rhythm Test

This test, part of the Seashore Test of Musical Talent, has also been an integral aspect of the Halstead-Reitan battery[102] and many of its derivatives. It requires the patient to discriminate between pairs of taperecorded musical tones that are either identical or different. The Seashore Rhythm Test is primarily used to assess right temporal lobe functioning, although impaired performance may result from more diffuse lesions.[10] Variable attentional levels, as well as difficulty in following directions, also adversely affect test performance, sometimes to the point of invalidating the results.

Speech Sounds Perception Test

This subtest of the Halstead-Reitan battery[100,101] requires the patient to indicate on an answer sheet which of four nonsense speechlike syllables he or she has heard via taperecorder headphones. The test includes 60 sets of syllables based on the vowel sound "ee" but beginning and ending with different consonants. It is an effective measure of sustained attention and has been consistently reported to be sensitive to the effects of brain damage, particularly left temporal lesions. The examiner must ensure that sufficient attention was maintained over the course of the administration to allow valid interpretation of the higher-level component of the test.

Tests of Tactile Perception

A variety of objective tests of tactile suppression, tactile recognition (stereognosis), and graphesthesia (e.g., fingertip writing, palm writing) have been developed to assess unilateral parietal lobe functioning. With the exception of normative data for objective comparison, they are very similar to the tests conducted during the standard neurologic and extended mental status examinations.

Tests of Visual Perception

It is crucial to establish the adequacy of the patient's visual acuity and visual perception and to rule out the possibility of unilateral neglect or inattention. Much of this is accomplished using clinical methods akin to the standard neurologic examination. Tests of neglect,[3] color vision,[59] visual recognition,[13] facial recognition,[13] fragmented visual stimuli,[77] and figure-ground discrimination[22,120] are merely examples of the many standardized tests and procedures that can be used to assess these functions. See Lezak[76] for a comprehensive review.

TESTS OF CONSTRUCTIONAL ABILITY

Bender Gestalt Test

The Bender Gestalt Test (originally the Bender Visual Motor Gestalt[9]) is a venerable, rapidly administered screening test of paper-and-pencil constructional ability. The patient reproduces each of nine geometric line-and-dot drawings. The design reproductions can be objectively scored for the errors of integration, distortion, perseveration, and rotation.[68] The designs are sufficiently simple that errorless performance is expected by age 12. The use of this test as a screen for organicity, unfortunately still a relatively common practice, is unwarranted given the current state of knowledge regarding brain-behavior relationships. However, its inclusion as a test of one type of constructional ability within a more comprehensive battery seems appropriate. It is sensitive to neurologic lesions in virtually all quadrants of the brain, especially in the nondominant hemisphere.[16] Golden[37] provides a thorough review of the advantages and disadvantages of this popular test.

Raven's Progressive Matrices

See page 199 for a discussion of this test, which is useful in assessing the visuospatial analytic component of the constructional process.

Benton Visual Retention Test

See page 196 for a review of this well-standardized test, which can be used to evaluate both reproduction constructional ability (design copying) and short-term recall reproduction (constructions from memory). The major advantages of this test are standard administration and scoring criteria, good normative data, and the availability of alternate, equivalent forms.

Minnesota Perception-Diagnostic Test

This copying test[35] is similar in approach to the Bender's Gestalt and Benton Visual Retention Tests. The test employs a design-copying format, with the reproductions being objectively scored for the degree of rotation. Normative data are provided for both adults and children.

Hooper Visual Organization Test

The Hooper Visual Organization Test (HVOT)[58] was originally developed to identify brain damage in hospitalized psychiatric patients but has more recently gained renewed favor in neuropsychology as a measure of visual analysis and organization and of the ability to synthesize disparate arts into a meaningful gestalt. It consists of 30 line drawings of relatively recognizable objects that have been cut into a variety of separate pieces. The patient must identify the target object by analyzing the set of object parts. The HVOT differs from similar puzzle construction measures by requiring no motor output, thus separating the visual perceptual component from the multifactor processes required in most constructional tasks. In addition to the patient's absolute level of performance (normal individuals typically miss no more than 5 of the 30 items), the HVOT is useful in demonstrating the nature of a patient's perceptual dysfunction. A number of researchers have demonstrated the Hooper's effectiveness in eliciting the perceptual fragmentation that can be seen in patients with right anterior lesions.[76]

Additional Tests of Constructional Ability

A wide range of clinical tests of construction have been used to supplement the more objectively scored and normed instruments. These include drawings to command (e.g., human figure drawing, bicycle drawing), geometric block constructions (e.g., WAIS-R Block Designs, Kohs Blocks, Grassi Block Substitution), puzzle completion (e.g., WAIS-R Objective Assembly), and stick and three-dimensional reproductions. See Benton and associates[13] and Lezak[76] for more complete reviews of these techniques.

TESTS OF VISUAL MOTOR SEQUENCING

Trail-Making Test

This test,[100] which is included in the Halstead-Reitan battery, has enjoyed continued popularity as a measure of visual searching, visual sequencing, perceptuomotor speed, and the ability to make alternating conceptual shifts efficiently. It is administered in two parts: Part A requires the patient to draw a line connecting 25 pseudorandomly numbered circles on a standard sheet of paper; Part B requires the patient to alternate between numbers and letters (i.e., 1-A-2-B-3 . . .) to connect the same number of circles. The patient is instructed to complete the tests "as rapidly but accurately as possible" because the score is the total time required to complete each part. Standard norms for various age groups are available,[23,56] as are a variety of data from specific clinical samples (e.g., Lewinson[75]). Research shows that this test is highly sensitive to the effects of brain dysfunction of any type and provides some equivocal indication that patients with frontal lobe lesions perform relatively more poorly.

Symbol Digit Modalities Test

This test[110] is an analog of the Digit Symbol and Coding subtests of the Wechsler series of intelligence tests, in that the patient is presented with a series of nine symbols, each associated with a number from 1 to 9. The patient then places as many numbers with the correct randomly ordered symbols as possible within a 90-second time period. The test can be administered with either a written or a verbal response, allowing a comparison of performance in each modality. Normative data are provided for age groups from 18 to 74, and for groups of differing educational levels and clinical diagnoses. The Symbol Digit Modalities Test requires sustained attention, visual searching, visual sequencing, and new-learning ability. The test is sensitive to deficits in any of these functions, as well as to brain dysfunction of many types.

TESTS OF MOTOR COORDINATION AND STRENGTH

Finger-Tapping Test

The Finger-Tapping Test,[100,102] also known as the Finger Oscillation Test, is a frequently used measure of fine motor coordination and speed. A variety of administrative methods have been published, all involving a number of tapping trials by the index finger of each hand and a mechanical or electrical recording tapping device. A number of reports suggest an average of approximately 55 ± 5 taps with the dominant hand during a 10-second trial and approximately 50 ± 4 taps with the nondominant hand. The test is fairly sensitive to brain dysfunction in general and, more specifically, to lesions in the area of the contralateral motor strip.[50]

Hand Dynamometer (Grip Strength)

The use of a mechanical hand dynamometer to assess grip strength over several trials with the right and left hands allows the accurate quantification of a common component of the standard neurologic examination. Standard norms are available from the many studies of the Halstead-Reitan battery and related literature.[56,114,117] Reductions in strength bilaterally when compared with the expected levels for age and sex, as well as disproportionate discrepancies between hands, may indicate brain dysfunction, particularly if peripheral factors are ruled out.

Tests of Lateral Dominance

Handedness has a close relationship to cerebral organization and thus is important in the interpretation of neuropsychologic results. The determination of handedness in clinical situations is often made by self-report. Although this simple method is sufficient for observably right-handed individuals, a more objective assessment technique should be used with reportedly left-handed and ambidextrous patients. A number of very similar observational checklists and rating scales are available.[76] Harris's Test of Lateral Dominance[52] includes both patient self-report for a variety of different activities and activities for observation (e.g., "Show me how you would kick a (foot)ball"). This test incorporates hand, foot, and eye dominance data. This can be useful, as there have been some suggestions that foot preference may be a more reliable index of cerebral dominance, in part because it is presumably less subject to cultural pressure.[107] Regardless of the technique used, the examiner should be able to determine the patient's dominance on the continuum from strongly right dominant to strongly left dominant, with special reference to the middle ground of ambidexterity.

Miscellaneous Motor Tests

In addition to these routinely administered tests, a wide variety of motor and motor-related instruments are available when more extensive testing of these functions is indicated. Among the more frequently used are the Porteus Maze Test,[92] the Luria Alternating Hand Series,[22] the Purdue Pegboard Test,[121] and the Grooved Pegboard Test.[84] See Anastasi[6] and Lezak[76] for descriptions of these tests and additional measures.

TESTS OF ACADEMIC ACHIEVEMENT

Peabody Individual Achievement Test–Revised

The Peabody Individual Achievement Test–Revised (PIAT-R)[79] measures reading recognition, comprehension, spelling, arithmetic, and general information in children and adults. It uses a multiple-choice format and is particularly useful when assessing the verbal but physically handicapped patient. It is not valid for evaluating patients with language problems; however it is especially useful in assessing patients who have a reading disorder. The test is well standardized and provides norms for age groups between 5.3 and 18.3 years.

Wide-Range Achievement Test–Revised

The Wide-Range Achievement Test–Revised (WRAT-R)[60] is probably the most frequently used objective test of achievement owing partly to its brevity. It assesses performance in reading recognition, spelling to dictation, and computational arithmetic. The test has been recently restandardized and is a useful clinical achievement test for both children and adults. A large-print version of the test protocol is available for use with patients who have deficient visual acuity.

Woodcock-Johnson Psychoeducational Battery–Revised: Tests of Achievement

The Woodcock-Johnson Psychoeducational Battery–Revised: Tests of Achievement (WJ-R-Ach)[127] represent a wide–age-range measure of academic achievement in the basic areas of reading, mathematics, and written language, as well as in basic science, social studies, and humanities. In neuropsychologic use, the three basic areas are most commonly used. A major advantage of this battery is the incorporation of supplemental subtests that allow the evaluation of specific deficits within the three basic areas. For example, reading cluster scores include measures of letter-word identification, word attack, passage comprehension and reading vocabulary. Similar achievement breakdowns are possible in mathematics and written language. Norms are provided for groups ranging from young children to elderly adults. The WJ-R-Ach is well developed psychometrically and well standardized; it offers a more comprehensive measure of academic functioning than most of the clinically useful achievement tests.[114]

PERSONALITY TESTS

Minnesota Multiphasic Personality Inventory–2

The recently revised Minnesota Multiphasic Personality Inventory–2 (MMPI-2)[53] continues to be the most commonly used standardized test of emotional status in both psychiatric and neurologic patients. The test consists of 567 statements about the patient's current functioning (e.g., "I am under a great deal of tension" and "It is safer to trust nobody"), to which the patient responds "true" or "false" as they apply to him or her. The protocol is scored either by hand using templates or by a readily available computer scoring program, with the resultant scale scores plotted on a graph that shows the patient's performance in the clinical areas of hypochondriasis, depression, hysteria, personality disorder, masculinity-femininity of interests, paranoia, psychasthenia (obsessive-compulsive), schizophrenia, hypomania, and social introversion. In addition to the ten basic clinical scales, the MMPI-2 provides 15 new content scales, offering a much more comprehensive description of the patient's emotional functioning.

The primary validity scales of L (lie or inconsistency of responses); F (significantly abnormal items atypically endorsed by normal individuals, suggesting an attempt to "fake bad," exaggeration, or frank psychopathology); and K (a suppressor variable reflecting social norm awareness, defensiveness, and attempts to "fake good") are obtained to help in judging the validity of test behavior. The MMPI-2 now includes several additional validity scales, as well as a breakdown of the patient's responses to test items having a high degree of face validity versus responses to items without a natural association with obvious psychologic distress. This allows an interpretation of the patient's tendency to exaggerate the degree of emotional distress, either consciously or unconsciously. In general, scores on validity and clinical scales more than two standard deviations above the mean are considered abnormal. A wide variety of interpretive guidebooks are available for general physicians, psychiatrists, and psychologists to aid in understanding the clinical significance of the patient's profile. There has been an increasing interest in the application of computer administration, scoring, and interpretation of this test.

At our current state of knowledge and experience with this technique, such an approach is more appropriate for normal and mildly abnormal psychiatric patients than for brain-damaged patients. The literature pertaining to the use of the MMPI with brain-damaged patients is expanding, with the reviews by Golden,[37] Golden and Vincente,[42] and Lezak[76] serving as useful introductions. See also Alfano and colleagues[5] for a recent study of its use in investigating the emotional changes that occur after closed head injury. The primary objection to use of the MMPI (and MMPI-2) with neurologic patients has been that such individuals may respond to MMPI items in the same way as patients having functional disorders, but for very different reasons. This is certainly a valid point, although the same objection can be raised for general medical patients, substance abusers, and a wide range of other clinical groups, as well as minority-group members. Certainly, all such potentially confounding factors should be considered when interpreting the MMPI-2 score of any patient. The MMPI-2 seems to be most useful in describing emotional functioning in neurologic patients, rather than in establishing a psychiatric diagnosis in accordance with the revised Diagnostic and Statistical Manual-III (DSM-III-R). Because of the recency of the introduction of the MMPI-2, investigations of its clinical use in neuropsychologic settings is only beginning. However, there is every reason to suggest that with some caution, the MMPI-2 should provide a reasonably objective picture of the emotional changes seen in some neurologic patients.

Other Personality Instruments

A variety of patient self-reporting scales of anxiety, depression, psychosocial pain, and social adjustment are available for those patients who are capable of responding validly. Such tests may be useful for assessing the subjective perception of emotional and social well-being, as well as for research. See Lezak,[76] Spreen and Strauss,[114] and Sweetland and Keyser[116] for more information regarding these instruments.

REFERENCES

1. Adams, KM: In search of Luria's battery: A false start. J Consult Clin Psychol 48:511, 1980.
2. Adams, RL and Tranton, SL: Development of a paper-and-pen form of the Halstead Category Test. J Consult Clin Psychol 49:298, 1981.
3. Albert, ML: A simple test of visual neglect. Neurology 23:658, 1973.
4. Albert, ML, et al: Clinical Aspects of Dysphasia. Springer-Verlag, New York, 1981.
5. Algano, DP, et al: The MMPI and closed-head injury. Clin Neuropsychol 6:134, 1992.
6. Anastasi, A: Psychological Testing, ed 5. Macmillan, New York, 1982.
7. Barona, A, Reynolds, CR and Chastain, R: A demographically based index of pre-morbid intelligence of the WAIS-R. J Consult Clin Psychol 52:885, 1984.
8. Baehr, ME and Corsini, RJ: The Press Test. London House Press, Park Ridge, IL, 1982.
9. Bender, L: Bender Motor Gestalt Test. American Orthopsychiatric Association, New York, 1946.
10. Beniak, TE: The assessment of cognitive deficits in uremia. Paper presented at the European meeting of the International Neuropsychological Society, Oxford, England, 1977.
11. Benton, AL: The Revised Visual Retention Test, ed 4. Psychological Corporation, New York, 1974.
12. Benton, AL and Hamsher, K: Multilingual Aphasia Examination. University of Iowa Press, Iowa City, 1978.
13. Benton, AL, et al: Contributions to Neuropsychological Assessment: A Clinical Manual. Oxford University Press, New York, 1983.
14. Berg, EA: A simple objective technique for measuring flexibility in thinking. J Gen Psychol 39:15–22, 1948.
15. Berg, R, Franzen, M, and Wedding, D: Screening for Brain Impairment. Springer Publishing, New York, 1987.
16. Black, FW and Bernard, B: Constructional apraxia as a function of lesion locus and size in patients with focal brain damage. Cortex 20:111, 1984.
17. Boll, TJ: The Halstead-Reitan neuropsychology battery. In Filskov, SB and Boll, TJ (eds): Handbook of Clinical Neuropsychology. Wiley-Interscience, New York, pp 577–607, 1981.
18. Bornstein, RA and Chelune, GJ: Factor Structure of the Wechsler Memory Scale—Revised. Clin Neuropsychol 2:107, 1988.
19. Browne, ER, Randt, CT, and Osborne, DP: Assessment of memory disturbances in aging. In Agnol, A, et al (eds): Aging, Vol 23, Aging Brain and Ergot Alkaloids. Raven Press, New York, pp 131–137, 1983.
20. Butler, M, Retzlaff, P, and Vanderploeg, R: Neuropsychological Test Usage. Prof Psychol Res Pract 22:510, 1991.
21. Calsyn, DA, O'Leary, MR, and Chaney, EF: Shortening the category test. J Consult Clin Psychol 48:788, 1980.
22. Christensen, AL: Luria's Neuropsychological Investigation, ed 2. Western Psychological Services, Los Angeles, 1979.
23. Davies, A: The influence of age on Trail Making Test performance. J Clin Psychol 24:96, 1968.
24. DeFilippus, NA and McCampbell, MS: The Booklet Category Test. Psychological Assessment Resources, Odessa, FL, 1980.

25. DeFilippus, NA and McCampbell, MS: The Booklet Category Test. Psychological Assessment Resources, New York, 1987.
26. Delise, DC and Kaplan, E: Hazards of a standardized neuropsychological test with low content validity: Comment on the Luria-Nebraska Neuropsychological Battery. J Consult Clin Psychol 51:396, 1983.
27. Delise, DC et al: California Verbal Learning Test. Psychological Corporation, New York, 1987.
28. DeRenzi, E and Faglioni, P: Normative data and screening power of a shortened version of the Token Test. Cortex 14:41, 1978.
29. Diller, L et al: Studies in cognition and rehabilitation in hemiplegia (rehabilitation monograph No. 50). New York University Medical Center Institute of Rehabilitation Medicine, New York, 1974.
30. Dodrill, CB: Sex differences on the Halstead-Reitan neuropsychological measures. J Clin Psychol 35:236, 1979.
31. Dunn, LM and Dunn, LM: Peabody Picture Vocabulary Test—Revised. American Guidance Service, Circle Pines, MN, 1981.
32. Elwood, RW: Factor Structure of the Wechsler Memory Scale—Revised (WMS-R) in a clinical sample: A methodological reappraisal. Clin Neuropsychol 5:329, 1991.
33. Fowler, RS: A simple non-language test for new learning. Percept Mot Skills 29:895, 1969.
34. Franzen, MD et al: Preliminary data concerning the test-retest and parallel forms reliability of the Randt Memory Test. Clin Neuropsychol 3:25, 1989.
35. Fuller, GB: Minnesota Perceptuo-Diagnostic Test (revised). Clinical Psychology Publishing, Brandon, VT, 1969.
36. Gates, AI and MacGinitie, WH: Gates-MacGinitie Reading Tests. Teachers College Press (Columbia), New York, 1969.
37. Golden, CJ: Clinical Interpretation of Objective Psychological Tests, ed 2. Allyn and Bacon, Needham Heights, MA, 1990.
38. Golden, CJ: Screening Test for the Luria-Nebraska Neuropsychological Battery: Adult and Children's Forms. Western Psychological Services, Los Angeles, 1987.
39. Golden, CJ: A standardized version of Luria's neuropsychological tests. In Filskov, SB and Boll, TJ (eds): Handbook of Clinical Neuropsychology. Wiley-Interscience, New York, pp 608–642, 1981.
40. Golden, CJ, Hammeke, TA, and Purisch, AD: Manual for the Luria-Nebraska Neuropsychological Battery. Western Psychological Services, Los Angeles, 1980.
41. Golden, CJ, Purisch, AD, and Hammeke, TA: Luria Nebraska Neuropsychological Battery: Forms I and II. Western Psychological Services, Los Angeles, 1986.
42. Golden, CJ and Vicente, PJ (eds): Foundations of Clinical Neuropsychology. Plenum, New York, 1983.
43. Goodglass, H and Kaplan, E: The Assessment of Aphasia and Related Disorders, ed 2. Lea & Febiger, Philadelphia, 1983.
44. Goodglass, H and Kaplan, E: The Assessment of Aphasia and Related Disorders, ed 2. Lea & Febiger, Philadelphia, 1987.
45. Gorham, DR: The Proverbs Test. Psychological Test Specialists, Missoula, MT, 1956.
46. Graham, FK and Kendall, BS: Memory-for-Designs Test: Revised general manual. Percept Mot Skills (Suppl)2-VIII;11:147, 1960.
47. Green RF and Martinez, JN (translators): Escala de Inteligencia Wechsler para adultos. Psychological Corporation, New York, 1968.
48. Gronwall, D: Advances in the assessment of attention and information processing after head injury. In Levin, H, et al: Neurobehavioral Recovery from Head Injury. Oxford University Press, New York, pp 355–371, 1987.
49. Gronwall, D and Sampson, H: The Psychological Effects of Concussion. Oxford University Press, Auckland, 1974.

50. Haaland, KY and Delaney, HD: Motor deficits after left or right hemisphere damage due to stroke or tumor. Neuropsychologia 19:17, 1981.
51. Halsted, W: Brain and Intelligence: A qualitative study of the frontal lobes. University of Chicago Press, Chicago, 1947.
52. Harris, AJ: Harris Tests of Lateral Dominance. Psychological Corporation, New York, 1958.
53. Hathaway, SR et al: Minnesota Multiphasic Personality Inventory–2: Manual for Administration and Scoring. University of Minnesota Press, Minneapolis, 1989.
54. Heaton, RK: Wisconsin Card Sorting Test Manual. Psychological Assessment Resources, Odessa, FL, 1981.
55. Heaton, RK, Baade, LE, and Johnson, KL: Neuropsychological tests results associated with psychiatric disorders in adult. Psychol Bull 85:141, 1978.
56. Heaton, RK, Grant, I, and Matthews, CG: Comprehensive norms for an expanded Halstead-Reitan Battery. Psychological Assessment Resources, Odessa, FL, 1991.
57. Holland, AL: Communicative Abilities in Daily Living. University Park Press, Baltimore, 1980.
58. Hooper, HE: The Hooper Visual Organization Test. Western Psychological Services, Los Angeles, 1958.
59. Ishihara, S: Tests for Color-Blindness. Kanehara Shuppan, Tokyo, 1964.
60. Jastak, S and Wilkinson, GS: The Wide Range Achievement Test (rev). Jastak Associates, Wilmington, DE, 1984.
61. Kaplan, E: WAIS-R as a Neuropsychological Instrument. Psychological Corporation, New York, 1991.
62. Kaplan, E, Goodglass, H, and Weintraub, S: Boston Naming Test. Lea & Febiger, Philadelphia, 1983.
63. Keenan, JS and Brassell, EG: Aphasia Language Performance Scales (ALPS). Pinnacle Press, Murfeesboro, TN, 1975.
64. Kertesz, A: Aphasia and Related Disorders: Taxonomy, Localization, and Recovery. Grune & Stratton, New York, 1979.
65. Kertesz, A: The Western Aphasia Battery. Grune & Stratton, New York, 1982.
66. Kimura, D: Right temporal-lobe damage: Perception of unfamiliar stimuli after damage. Arch Neurol 8:264, 1963.
67. Kimura, D and McGlone, J: Neuropsychology Test Procedures. DK Consultants, London, 1983.
68. Koppitz, EM: The Bender Gestalt Test for Young Children. Grune & Stratton, New York, 1964.
69. Lawson, JS, Inglis, J, and Stroud, TWF: A laterality index of cognitive impairment derived from a principal components analysis of the WAIS-R. J Consult Clin Psychol 51:841, 1983.
70. Leiter, RG: Examiner's Manual for the Leiter International Performance Scale. Stoelting, Chicago, 1969.
71. Leiter, RG: General Instructions for the Leiter International Performance Scale. Western Psychological Services, Los Angeles, 1976.
72. Levin, HS, Eisenberg, HM, and Benton, AL: Mild Head Injury. Oxford University Press, New York, 1989.
73. Levin, HS, Grafman, J, and Eisenberg, HM: Neurobehavioral Recovery from Head Injury. Oxford University Press, New York, 1987.
74. Levine, MN: Leiter International Performance Scale: A Handbook. Western Psychological Services, Los Angeles, 1982.
75. Lewinson, PM: Psychological assessment of patients with brain injury. Unpublished manuscript. University of Oregon, Eugene, OR, 1973.
76. Lezak, MD: Neuropsychological Assessment. Oxford University Press, New York, 1983.
77. Likert, R and Quasha, WH: The Revised Minnesota Paper Form Board Test. Psychological Corporation, New York, 1970.

78. Loring, DJ: The Wechsler Memory Scale—Revised, or the Wechsler Memory Scale—Revisited? Clin Neuropsychol 3:59, 1989.
79. Markwardt, FC: Peabody Individual Achievement Test—Revised. American Guidance Services, Circle Pines, MN, 1989.
80. Marsh, GG and Hirsch, SH: Effectiveness of two tests of visual retention. J Clin Psychol 38:115, 1982.
81. Matarazzo, JD: Psychological assessment versus psychological testing. Am Psychol 45:999, 1990.
82. Matarazzo, JD: Wechsler's Measurement and Appraisal of Adult Intelligence, ed 5. Oxford University Press, New York, 1972.
83. Matthews, CG: Neuropsychology practice in a hospital setting. In Filskov, SB and Boll, TJ (eds): Handbook of Clinical Neuropsychology. Wiley-Interscience, New York, pp 645–685, 1981.
84. Matthews, CG and Klovc, H: Instruction Manual for the Adult Neuropsychology Test Battery. University of Wisconsin Medical School, Madison, WI, 1964.
85. Melendez, F: The Adult Neuropsychological Questionnaire (ANQ). Psychological Assessment Resources, Odessa, FL, 1978.
86. Mesulam, M-M: Principles of Behavioral Neurology. FA Davis, Philadelphia, 1985.
86a. Mesulam, M-M: Principles of Behavioral Neurology: Tests of Directed Attention and Memory. FA Davis Company, Philadelphia, 1985.
87. Moran, LJ and Mefferd, RB: Repetitive psychometric measures. Psychol Rep 5:269, 1959.
88. O'Donnell, WE, DeSoto, CB, and Reynolds, DMcQ: Sensitivity and specificity of the Neuropsychological Impairment Scale (NIS). J Clin Psychol 40:553, 1984.
89. O'Donnell, WE, Reynolds, DMcQ, and DeSoto, CB: Validity and reliability of the Neuropsychological Impairment Scale (NIS). J Clin Psychol 40:549, 1984.
90. O'Donnell, WE and Reynolds, DMcQ: Neuropsychological Impairment Scale. Unpublished Manual, Annapolis, MD, 1983.
91. Porch, BE: Porch Index of Communicative Ability. Consulting Psychologists Press, Palo Alto, CA, 1967.
92. Porteus, SD: Porteus Maze Test. Psychological Corporation, New York, 1965.
93. Preston, J: Neuropsychological Screening Exam. Wilmington Press, Dallas, 1983.
94. Psychological Assessment Resources: Neuropsychological Status Examination. Psychological Assessment Resources, Odessa, FL, 1983.
95. Randt, CT and Brown, ER: Administration Manual: Randt Memory Test. Life Science Associates, Bayport, NY, 1983.
96. Randt, CT, Brown, ER, and Osborne, DP: A memory test for longitudinal measurement of mild to moderate deficits. Clin Neuropsychol II;4:184, 1980.
97. Raven, JC: Guide to the standard progressive matrices. Psychological Corporation, New York, 1977.
98. Raven, JC: Guide to using the coloured progressive matrices. Psychological Corporation, New York, 1977.
99. Raven, JC: The Advanced Progressive Matrices. Psychological Corporation, New York, 1977.
100. Reitan, R: Investigation of the validity of Halstead's measures of biological intelligence. Arch Neurol Psychiatry 48:475, 1955.
101. Reitan, R: A research program on the psychological effects of brain lesions in human beings. In Ellis, N (ed): International Review of Research in Mental Retardation, Vol 1. Academic Press, New York, pp 153–218, 1966.
102. Reitan, R and Davison, LA: Clinical Neuropsychology: Current Status and Applications. Hemisphere, New York, 1974.
103. Rey, A: L'exam clinique en psychologie. Presses Universitaires de France, Paris, 1964.
104. Roman, DD, et al: Extended norms for the Paced Serial Addition Test. The Clinical Neuropsychologist 5:33, 1991.

105. Russell, EW, Neuringer, C, and Goldstein, G: Assessment of Brain Damage: A Neuropsychological Key Approach. Wiley-Interscience, New York, 1970.

106. Ryan, JJ and Paolo, AM: A screening procedure for estimating premorbid intelligence in the elderly. Clin Neuropsychol 6:53, 1992.

107. Searleman, AA: Subject variables and cerebral organization for language. Cortex 16:239, 1980.

108. Shipley, WC: Institute of Living Scale. Western Psychological Services, Los Angeles, 1946.

109. Smith, A: Dominant and nondominant hemispherectomy. In Smith, WL (ed): Drugs, Development and Cerebral Function. Charles C Thomas, Springfield, IL, pp 37–68, 1972.

110. Smith, A: Symbol Digit Modalities Test Manual. Western Psychological Services, Los Angeles, 1973.

111. Spiers, PA: The Luria-Nebraska Neuropsychological Battery revisited: A theory in practice or just practicing. J Consult Clin Psychol 50:301, 1982.

112. Spreen, O and Benton, AL: Sentence Repetition Test. University of Victoria Neuropsychology Laboratory, Victoria, BC, 1969.

113. Spreen, O and Benton, AL: Neurosensory Center Comprehensive Examination for Aphasia. University of Victoria Neuropsychology Laboratory, Victoria, BC, 1969.

114. Spreen, O and Strauss, E: A Compendium of Neuropsychological Tests. Oxford University Press, New York, 1991.

115. Stambrook, M: The Luria-Nebraska Neuropsychological Battery: A promise that may be partly fulfilled. J Clin Neuropsychol 5:247, 1983.

116. Sweetland, RC and Keyser, DJ (eds): Tests. Test Corporation of America, Kansas City, Missouri, 1983.

117. Swiercinsky, D: Manual for the Adult Neuropsychological Evaluation. Charles C Thomas, Springfield, IL, 1978.

118. Talland, GA: Deranged Memory. Academic Press, New York, 1965.

119. Thorndike, RL, Hagen, EP, and Sattler, JM: Stanford-Binet Intelligence Scale, ed 4. Riverside Publishing, Chicago, 1986.

120. Thurstone, LL: A Factorial Study of Perception. University of Chicago Press, Chicago, 1944.

121. Tiffin, J: Purdue Pegboard Test. Science Research Association, Chicago, 1948.

122. Tites, RL: Neuropsychological Test Manual. Royal Ottawa Hospital, Ottawa, Ontario, 1977.

123. Wechsler, D: The Wechsler Intelligence Scale for Children–III. Psychological Corporation, New York, 1991.

124. Wechsler, D: Wechsler Memory Scale—Revised. Psychological Corporation, New York, 1987.

125. Wechsler, D: Wechsler Adult Intelligence Scale—Revised (WAIS-R). Psychological Corporation, New York, 1981.

126. Williams, MJ: Memory Assessment Scales (MAS). Psychological Assessment Resources. Odessa, FL, 1991.

127. Woodcock, RW and Mather, N: Woodcock-Johnson Tests of Achievement. DLM Teaching Resources, Allen, Texas, 1989.

128. Wysocki, JJ and Sweet, JJ: Identification of brain-damaged, schizophrenic, and normal medical patients using a brief neuropsychological screening battery. Int J Clin Neuropsychol 7:40, 1985.

129. Zachary, RA: Shipley Institute of Living Scale—Revised Manual. Western Psychological Services, Los Angeles, 1986.

Appendix 2

Mental Status Examination Recording Form

PATIENT INFORMATION

Patient name: Date:
Address: Case #:

Phone: Hospital #:
Date of birth: Place of birth:
Age: Sex:
Education:
    Highest level: Age at completion:
    Failures or honors:
Handedness:
    Patient: Family:
Occupation:
Medical diagnosis:
    Onset and nature:

Hemiplegia:
    (Circle)   None   Recovered   Right   Left

Hemianopia:
    (Circle)   None   Recovered   Right   Left

Neurosurgical information:

Electroencephalograph (EEG) focus:

MRI, CT scan, brain scan, angiogram, and so forth:

(Starred items are essential and should be used with all patients.)
*I.   Behavioral Observations

    *A. History of behavior change, memory difficulties, bizarre behavior, change in work habits, and the like:

*B. Physical Appearance:

*C. Emotional Status (e.g., confusion, depression, anxiety, lability):

D. Frontal Lobe Test Results (see related cortical functions):

*E. Denial or Neglect:

*II. Level of Consciousness

    *A. Rate: Alert_____ Lethargic_____ Stupor_____ Coma_____

    *B. Describe stimulus necessary to arouse patient, and record patient's response:

*III. Attention

    *A. Observation of patient during examination:
    *B. Digit repetition: Repeat digits at a rate of one per second.

ITEM	CHECK IF CORRECT
3-7	_____
2-4-9	_____
8-5-2-7	_____
2-9-6-8-3	_____
5-7-1-9-4-6	_____
8-1-5-9-3-6-2	_____
3-9-8-2-5-1-4-7	_____
7-2-8-5-4-6-7-3-9	_____

C. Vigilance: Repeat letters at a rate of one per second. Tell patient to indicate by tapping the table whenever he or she hears the letter "A."

```
L  T  P  E  A  O  A  I  C  T  D  A  L  A  A
A  N  I  A  B  F  S  A  M  R  Z  E  O  A  D
P  A  K  L  A  U  C  J  T  O  E  A  B  A  A
Z  Y  F  M  U  S  A  H  E  V  A  A  R  A  T
```

1. Errors of omission: _____

2. Errors of commission: _____

D. Unilateral inattention:

*IV. Language

    *A. Spontaneous speech:

        *1. Describe, including fluency, articulation, and presence of paraphasias:

        2. Verbal fluency: Total words: _____

                        Total animals: _____

    *B. Comprehension:

        *1. Patient's response to pointing commands:
Ask patient to point to one, two, three, then four room objects or body parts in sequence. Record adequacy of performance.

        *2. Patient's response to yes-no questions:
(e.g., "Is it raining today?" or "Is Grant still president?")

    *C. Repetition:

Tell the patient to repeat each of the following:

ITEM	CHECK IF CORRECT
1. Ball	_____
2. Help	_____
3. Airplane	_____
4. Hospital	_____
5. Mississippi River	_____
6. The little boy went home.	_____
7. We all went over there together.	_____
8. The old car wouldn't start on Tuesday morning.	_____
9. The short fat boy dropped the china vase.	_____
10. Each fight readied the boxer for the championship bout.	_____

*D. Naming and Word Finding:

Tell the patient to name the following simple colors and objects:

ITEM	CHECK IF CORRECT
1. Colors	
a. Red	_____
b. Blue	_____
c. Yellow	_____
d. Pink	_____
e. Purple	_____
2. Body parts	
a. Eye	_____
b. Leg	_____
c. Teeth	_____
d. Thumb	_____
e. Knuckles	_____
3. Clothing and room objects	
a. Door	_____
b. Watch	_____
c. Shoe	_____
d. Shirt	_____
e. Ceiling	_____
4. Parts of objects	
a. Watch stem (winder)	_____
b. Coat lapel	_____
c. Watch crystal	_____
d. Sole of shoe	_____
e. Buckle of belt	_____

E. Reading:

Describe level of adequacy (words, sentences, paragraphs) and note types of errors:

F. Writing:

Describe level of adequacy and note types of errors:

G. Spelling:

Describe performance to dictation and note errors:

*V. Memory: Most of the following memory tasks evaluate verbal memory. In patients with language disturbance (aphasia), the visual memory tests must be used.

    *A. Immediate Recall (short-term memory):
        Refer to Digit Repetition in Section III.

    *B. Orientation:

CHECK IF CORRECT

        *1. Person
            a. Name   _____
            b. Age   _____
            c. Birth date   _____
        *2. Place
            a. Location (at present)   _____
            b. City location   _____
            c. Home address   _____
        *3. Time
            a. Date   _____
            b. Day of the week   _____
            c. Time of day   _____
            d. Season of the year   _____
            e. Duration of time with   _____
                examiner

    *C. Remote Memory:

**CHECK IF CORRECT
OR ADEQUATE**

        *1. Personal Information
            a. Where were you born?   _____
            b. School information   _____
            c. Vocational history   _____
            d. Family information   _____

        *2. Historic Facts
            a. Four US presidents during   _____
                your lifetime
            b. Last war   _____

    *D. New-Learning Ability:
        Tell the patient, "I am going to tell you four words, which I want you to remember." Have the patient repeat the four words after they are initially presented and then say that you will ask him or her to remember the words later.

Continue with the examination, and at intervals of 5, 10, and 30 minutes, ask the patient to recall the words. Use categoric ("one word is a color") or phonemic ("one word begins with B") cues if he or she is unable to recall the word spontaneously on any trial. Record the type and amount of cuing necessary. Two alternate sets of words are provided.

1. Four Unrelated Words

	5 min	10 min	30 min
a. Brown (Fun)	———	———	———
b. Honesty (Loyalty)	———	———	———
c. Tulip (Carrot)	———	———	———
d. Eyedropper (Ankle)	———	———	———

Describe type of cues used if necessary:

2. Verbal Story for Immediate Recall:
   Tell the patient, "I am going to read you a short story, which I want you to remember. Listen closely to what I read because I will ask you to tell me the story when I finish." Read the story slowly and carefully, but without pausing at the slash marks. After completing the paragraph, tell the patient to retell the story as accurately as possible. Record the number of correct memories (information within the slashes) and describe confabulation if it is present.

   It was July / and the Rogers / had packed up / their four children / in the station wagon / and were off / on vacation.

   They were taking / their yearly trip / to the beach / at Gulf Shores.

   This year / they were making / a special / one-day stop / at the Aquarium / in New Orleans.

   After a long day's drive / they arrived / at the motel / only to discover / that in their excitement / they had left / the twins / and their suitcases / in the front yard.

   a. Number of correct memories: _____
   b. Describe confabulation if present:

3. Visual Memory (hidden objects):
   Tell the patient that you are going to hide some objects around the office, desk, or bed and that you want him

or her to remember where they are. Hide four or five common objects (e.g., keys, pen, reflex hammer) in various areas in the patient's sight. After a delay of several minutes, ask the patient to find the objects. Ask patient to name those items he or she is unable to find.

a. Number of hidden objects found: _____
b. Number of hidden objects named but not found: _____
c. Number of locations indicated but objects not named: _____

*4. Visual Memory (visual design reproduction):
            (see stimulus cards)

ITEM	**SCORE**
a. Design 1	_____
b. Design 2	_____
c. Design 3	_____
d. Design 4	_____

    Total score: _____

5. Paired Associated Learning:
    Tell the patient that you are going to read a list of words two at a time. The patient will be expected to remember the words that go together (e.g., big—little). When he or she is clear as to the directions, read the first list of words at the rate of one pair per second. After reading the first list, test for recall by presenting the first recall list. Give the first word of a pair and ask for the word that went with it. Correct incorrect responses and proceed to the next pair. After the first recall has been completed, allow a 10-second delay and continue with the second presentation and recall lists.

PRESENTATION LISTS

1	2
a. Weather—Bag	a. House—Income
b. High—Low	b. Weather—Bag
c. House—Income	c. Book—Page
d. Book—Page	d. High—Low

RECALL LISTS

1	2
a. House _____	a. High _____
b. High _____	b. House _____

c. Weather _____   c. Book _____
d. Book _____   d. Weather _____

1. Number of easy paired associates recalled: _____
2. Number of difficult paired associates recalled: _____

*VI. Constructional Ability

*A. Reproduction drawings:
Ask the patient to copy the following drawings in the space provided.

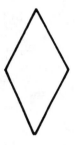

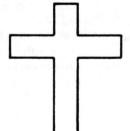

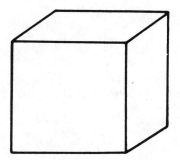

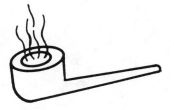

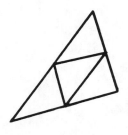

ITEM	SCORE
1. Vertical diamond	_____
2. Two-dimensional cross	_____
3. Three-dimensional cube	_____
4. Three-dimensional pipe	_____
5. Triangle within a triangle	_____

Total score: _____

*B. Drawings to Command:
Tell the patient to draw the following pictures in the space provided.

Clock with all numbers

Daisy in flowerpot

House in perspective

ITEM	SCORE
1. Clock	_____
2. Daisy in flowerpot	_____
3. House in perspective	_____

Total score: _____

C. Block Designs:

(See stimulus cards)

ITEM	SCORE
1. Design 1	_____
2. Design 2	_____
3. Design 3	_____
4. Design 4	_____

Total score: _____

Describe types of errors:

*VII. Higher Cognitive Functions

A. Fund of Information:

ITEM	CHECK IF CORRECT
1. How many weeks are in a year?	_____
2. Why do people have lungs?	_____

3. Name four US Presidents since 1940.   _____

4. Where is Denmark?   _____

5. How far is it from New York to Los Angeles?   _____

6. Why are light colored clothes cooler in the summer than dark colored clothes?   _____

7. What is the capital of Spain?   _____

8. What causes rust?   _____

9. Who wrote the Odyssey?   _____

10. What is the Acropolis?   _____

Total score: _____

*B. Calculations:

Describe the patient's adequacy in performance and types of errors made on the following types of calculations:

1. Verbal rote examples:

a. Addition $(4 + 6)$
b. Subtraction $(8 - 5)$
c. Multiplication (2×8)
d. Division $(56 \div 8)$

2. Verbal complex examples:

a. Addition $(14 + 17)$
b. Subtraction $(43 - 38)$
c. Multiplication (21×5)
d. Division $(128 \div 8)$

*3. Written complex examples:

a. Addition $\begin{array}{r} 108 \\ + 79 \end{array}$

b. Subtraction $\begin{array}{r} 605 \\ - 86 \end{array}$

c. Multiplication $\begin{array}{r} 108 \\ \times 36 \end{array}$

d. Division $43\overline{)559}$

*C. Proverb Interpretation:
   Tell the patient to explain the following sayings. Record the
   answers.

	ITEM	**SCORE**
1.	Don't cry over spilled milk.	_____
2.	Rome wasn't built in a day.	_____
3.	A drowning man will clutch at a straw.	_____
4.	A golden hammer breaks an iron door.	_____
5.	The hot coal burns; the cold one blackens.	_____

   Total score: _____
   Total concrete responses: _____

*D. Similarities

ITEM	**SCORE**
1. Turnip............................Cauliflower	_____
2. Car..Airplane	_____
3. Desk..................................Bookcase	_____
4. Poem..Novel	_____
5. Horse......................................Apple	_____

   Total score: _____
   Total concrete responses: _____

E. Conceptual Series Completion:

ITEM	**CHECK IF CORRECT**
1. A B C D ____	_____
2. 1 4 7 10 ____ ____	_____
3. AZ BY CX D ____	_____
4. tote to snow on spun up stab ____ ____	_____
5. elephant 87654321 plan 5732 lap ____ ____ ____	_____

   Total score: _____

VIII. Related Cortical Functions

    A. Ideomotor Apraxia:

    Describe the adequacy of the patient's performance in carrying out motor acts to command using buccofacial, limb, and whole body commands. Indicate if imitation or use of the real object was necessary to facilitate performance.

ITEM	SCORE
1. Blow out a match.	_____
2. Drink through a straw.	_____
3. Lick crumbs off your lips.	_____
4. Comb your hair.	_____
5. Flip a coin.	_____

    B. Ideational Apraxia:

    Describe the adequacy of the patient's performance on the following complex motor tasks:

        1. Letter-envelope-stamp
        2. Candle-holder-match
        3. Toothpaste-toothbrush

    C. Right-Left Disorientation:

ITEM	CHECK IF CORRECT
1. Identification on self	_____
a. Show me your right foot	_____
b. Show me your left hand	_____
2. Crossed commands on self	_____
a. With your right hand touch your left shoulder.	_____
b. With your left hand touch your right ear.	_____
3. Identification on examiner	_____
a. Point to my left knee.	_____
b. Point to my right elbow.	_____
4. Crossed commands on examiner	_____
a. With your right hand point to my left eye.	_____
b. With your left hand point to my left foot.	_____

Describe nature and degree of errors made:

D. Finger Agnosia:
Describe the adequacy of the patient's nonverbal and verbal
performance.

E. Gerstmann's Syndrome:
Describe the nature and degree of impairment in the
following areas if present in the patient:

   1. Finger agnosia: _____
   2. Right-left disorientation: _____
   3. Dysgraphia: _____
   4. Dyscalculia: _____

F. Visual Agnosia:
Describe any deficits in visual identification of objects,
naming of objects whose use can be demonstrated, color
naming, and facial recognition:

G. Astereognosis:
Describe deficits:

Left hand _____
Right hand _____

H. Geographic Disorientation:
   1. Describe evidence of disorientation obtained from
      history:

   2. Map localization:

      Describe patient's ability to localize well-known cities on
      a map:

   3. Orientation of self in hospital:

      Describe patient's ability to orient self within the hospital
      environment:

*I. Denial and Neglect:
If present, describe patient's response.

	YES	NO
1. Does patient frankly deny his illness?	——	——
2. Is there evidence of unilateral neglect? (e.g., shaving one side of face, dressing one arm, and so on)	——	——
3. Is there evidence of unilateral neglect on drawings? (e.g., absence of numbers on one side of clock or absence of one side of picture)	——	——

J. Frontal Lobe Tests:

1. Drawings:
Tell the patient to copy and continue the following sequence. Record evidence of perseveration or loss of sequence.

2. Alternating hand sequences:
This is a motor alternation task that uses both hands. Initially, the patient places both hands on the desk, one in a fist and one with the fingers extended palm down. Tell the patient to alternate the position of the two hands rapidly (simultaneously extending the fingers of one hand while making a fist with the other). Record if the patient is unable to maintain the alternating sequence.

SUMMARY OF FINDINGS

1. Describe major areas of impairment:

2. Tentative neurobehavioral diagnosis:

3. Tentative localization:

4. Tentative clinical diagnosis:

5. Proposed management plans:

Index

An "F" following a page number indicates a figure; a "T" following a page number indicates a table.